THE SPIRIT OF THE HORSE

*Finding Healing and Spiritual Connection
with the Horse*

PAM BILLINGE

blackbird

First Published in 2021
This edition published in 2022
Blackbird Digital Books
2/25 Earls Terrace
London W8 6LP
www.blackbird-books.com
Copyright © Pam Billinge 2021
Pam Billinge has asserted her right to be identified as the author of this work.
A CIP catalogue record for this book is available from the British Library
ISBN 9781838278663
Cover design by Germancreative

About the Author

Pam Billinge is a therapist, coach and author who specialises in embodied horse-led learning. This unique approach relies entirely on the emergent relational process between horse and human. At her bases in the UK and in France, Pam supports people of all nationalities, ages and walks of life with their personal and professional development. Through her workshops and her writing Pam wishes to share the healing wisdom of horses whilst advancing the cause of this sometimes misunderstood species. She hopes also through her work to reconnect us with the natural world from which we are too often separated.

Also by Pam Billinge

THE SPELL OF THE HORSE

Stories of healing and personal transformation with nature's finest teachers

When Pam's mother was diagnosed with terminal cancer, she began to notice the way her horse responded to her emotional turmoil. Thus began an exploration into the spiritual relationship between horses and humans and their infinite capacity to help us heal. By sharing her own path to redemption through personal tragedy, and other stories of healing inspired by the incredible interactions she has observed between horse and human, Pam puts forward her uplifting insights about the true nature of the horse, setting out some simple principles to help the reader transcend life's challenges.

In praise of The Spell of the Horse

'Honest, authentic and full of wisdom.' Goodreads

'Beautifully-written, finely-constructed, humanely-told. I have read (and written) many books about leadership development, and this is one of the best.' Jonathan Gosling, Emeritus Professor of Leadership, University of Exeter and Director of Pelumbra Ltd

'This book will repay the few hours it will take you to read it many times over.' Goodreads

'Not just for horse lovers but for anyone interested in finding sustainable ways to overcome personal challenges.' Goodreads

'Pam Billinge writes with a wonderful beauty.' Liz Loves Books

'Having spent several years training as a counsellor, I have learnt more about the human mind and spirit from just reading this book.' Amazon reader

'Her special affinity and deep respect for horses shines through with every well-written word and every emotional connection.' Jaffa Reads Too

For Dee and Jenny
And for you, the reader

Contents

Introduction

The promises

In 2008, a small brown Quarter Horse called Coop changed my life. Lost and anxious after a destructive marriage, divorce, redundancy and multiple bereavements, I needed to get away. I signed up for an intensive two-month course in Colorado's Rocky Mountains to learn natural ways of interfacing with horses. Coop reconnected me to myself in the most affirmatory way possible. I learned how to be fully in the moment, to let go of fear and to dare to dream. The way in which I saw horses, my work as a therapist and coach, and indeed myself, were changed forever. I write about this transformational experience in *The Spell of the Horse*.

In my final days at the ranch I made myself two promises. The first, that I would find a way of integrating the healing power of horses into my work as a psychotherapist and a leadership coach. I had no idea how I would do it, with no facilities to work at and only one horse at home in my 'herd'. Yet excitement bubbled under my skin in a way it had never done before. However crazy it seemed I knew this was what I must do. I vowed I would find a way – if one horse could change me so much, then why would others not be able to do the same for my clients?

The second part of my vow was that I would one day have my horse, or horses, living with me at home. Since I bought my first, Delilah, 18 years earlier, I had always been obliged to use livery yards. If I was lucky, my horse would be a few miles away from home, but sometimes they were much further. I

1

fitted into someone else's rules and decisions about their care, and tolerated the fallings out and judgemental opinions of my human stable-mates. In Colorado I lived alongside Coop for 6 weeks, lodged in a log cabin a stone's throw from where he was kept. I had come to know the closeness which is possible when sharing the same space and interacting throughout the days. Being a daily visitor to my horse on someone else's terms didn't feel enough anymore.

The great surprise was that it was the first of my commitments which had been the easiest to manifest. Within a year of returning from my adventure in the mountains I was running successful leadership development programmes for my corporate clients centred around experiential interaction with a herd. I was also offering horse-led psychotherapy to private clients of all ages and walks of life. (I describe what I do as being 'horse-led' rather than 'equine assisted' because I feel it is I who assist the horses in their healing work, not the other way around.)

As this business grew, I developed a collaboration with a farm based in Wiltshire to host programmes and formed a team of like-minded professionals around me. The materialisation of this collective seemed almost miraculous such was the synchronicity of events. There was an indisputable 'rightness' to the enterprise. Changes in my personal circumstances left me needing a new base, so I relocated to a beautiful county in South West England to make my home and start afresh.

Wiltshire immediately felt like the right place for me to be. But with land prices beyond my reach the second promise faded into a daydream, gathering dust on the 'if only' shelf. When in idle moments I browsed the internet looking at equestrian properties which I *could* afford, in far-flung parts of the United Kingdom or in France, it was with the longing of a window shopper who feels she will never be able to step into the shop. It was the same feeling I used to have as a child when

2

I would ask my parents for a pony, knowing that they would never buy me one. My mum would always say kindly, 'Yes of course you can have one ... one day ... when we are rich.' And I got used to that day never coming.

Being able to see my herd from the garden, being able to create an environment for their optimum health, whilst building a therapeutic workspace which suited the way I wanted to welcome my clients – all this became a fantasy. I stopped believing that it would be possible, at least for me.

Don't stop believing

These patterns which we grow up with, whether it is expecting that you will never have what you long for, that you are not good enough to deserve it, or that you will fail so it is better not to try, stay with us into our adult lives without us even realising it. We receive in life what we expect to receive, and these often-undetected belief systems limit our ability to be happy.

The important thing to understand is that if your dream doesn't go away, if it still beckons from the shelf you have put it on, then it is more than a wistful fancy and you close your ears at your peril.

And this promise of mine, it did keep calling. *The Spirit of the Horse* tells the story of where it took me, what I learned and am still learning on that path – about myself, the profound nature of horses and about life, love and leadership.

Along the way I have worked with many inspiring people. They have often left me wiser and always left me feeling blessed. I thank them for trusting me and my horses to walk beside them for a little while. I share, too, some of their stories with you. To protect their anonymity identities have been fictionalised, but what happened between the person and the horses are just as described. Individuals whose personal stories are featured have given permission for, and many have contributed to, the narrative.

You may be a horse-lover who simply wants to lose yourself in the deep affection for the species which lives in these pages. You may be asking questions about the nature of your relationship with your own horse or be interested to learn about my professional approach. You may not know horses at all, but are exploring our bindings to nature and how it might save us, the human race, from ourselves. Or perhaps you are a business person, parent, teacher or spouse looking for new ways to love and lead those for whom you are responsible. For whatever reason you come to *The Spirit of the Horse*, know that I held you in my mind when I wrote it. I created this book, which soon I will set free to find its way to you, for the joy of sharing the many gifts which my life yields. It is a privilege and pleasure to be a small part of your journey, and I am grateful to you for inviting me in.

PART ONE

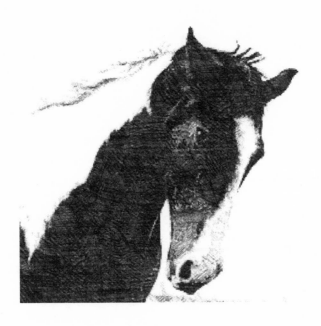

1

Moonlight Escape

Late October 2018

The lorry had been left a quarter of a mile up the rural track to facilitate a nocturnal departure. In the full moonlight the autumnal canopy running its length shone in sepia tones and the stones beneath my feet glistened. It was so bright I didn't need the torch bulging in my pocket. The horse transporter and his assistant were already at the gate waiting for me to arrive with the key. I wasn't sure if I was relieved or not to see them. In some way I hoped that I would have time on my own with the herd to ask them once again if I was doing the right thing. I wasn't sure if I would bitterly regret this one day or be eternally grateful.

The three horses were more than surprised to see us emerge from the shadows at 2am that October morning. I had no time to reconsider my decision or say a silent goodbye to this beauty spot and the memories it held. The transporters were cheerful, efficient, swift. They didn't say much which was just as well because I couldn't have spoken through the wad of emotion in my throat. Before I knew it the doors of the large lorry were creaking shut with the horses inside. This chapter in my life was closing, the next had not yet begun.

2

The White Horse Watches Over

December 2012

The incessant rain forced me into my car rather than my walking boots to go out exploring. Gingerly I drove, the water lying on every bend concealed potholes and soft verges which I knew could really spoil my day. And then, teetering over the crest of the single-lane humped-back bridge, I saw it. A huge prancing equine figure, dug into the hillside, rising before me.

I had seen pictures of the various chalk horses which adorned the rolling downs in this part of the country but I had not realised that there was one so close by. This turf carving had graced the Pewsey Vale for two hundred years, emblematic of the tranquility which oozed from the landscape. Commissioned by a Victorian landowner it was not archaeologically significant in itself, but it piaffed on the site of a Neolithic long barrow, guarding the souls who had walked there four thousand years before.

A new home

A failed relationship and a year of grief following the unexpected death of my older brother had set me adrift. I needed to throw down an anchor and chose this verdant corner of South West England, known for its ancient history, pagan roots and swathes of hill and heathland. I had the beginnings of a network in the area to support my transition and a venue where I would be able to develop my horse-led learning business. What did I have to lose?

I settled in a hamlet a few miles from the great white horse which seemed to have called me that day. I bought a small house which with love would become pretty. When I heard of a field coming up for rent a mile away I made sure that I became the next tenant. My herd of four, Winston, Ruby, Dawn and Ellie, would dwell in the heart of this exquisite vale, watched over from afar by their symbolic counterpart.

To access the field where the horses were soon installed involved a long walk along a track. It was lined with hedge and copse, stony in some places and muddy in others. It took me away from the village into farmland abundant with wildlife. In March there was enough wild garlic to keep me in pesto for a year and in September there were blackberries for jam. Occasionally walkers passed along the footpath but most days I would be alone there with the herd. It was a place where I would find healing, quietude and space, where melancholy dispersed and appreciation took its place. For the first time since I had owned horses I was able to create an environment which I didn't need to share and soon this five-acre field became an extension of my home.

Belonging

In the Liverpool suburb where I was raised neighbours often visited each other uninvited, sometimes even in their slippers, whether to drink tea, feed pets or monitor children. It had taken me a long time to grow used to the privacy (or might I say distance) maintained in other places I had lived. Over the years there had been few of my neighbours I could have called friends.

But here under the eye of the White Horse it was different. I found a bag full of home-grown lettuce leaves on my step. A jar of marmalade followed, then runner beans and soon an invitation to a Meet your Neighbours gathering. This was a locality with heart and in the following months I was enfolded within it. Companions came forward for dog-walks, rides, shared meals and drinks. Lifts were offered when cars broke down and shovels emerged when the snow fell. Here I felt looked after. There was a giving and taking of care founded on common humanity and kindness. This was a place I felt safe. 'Here I will stay' I vowed quietly to myself. Why would I ever leave?

3

Zeus

There was something indescribably ancient about the dark brown dappled pony. It was as if, around him, a space opened up in which time no longer passed sequentially but simultaneously. Through him, an energy of the horses of six million years pulsed. I couldn't even describe it as wildness, although he was of feral stock. There was nobility, grace, wisdom, solidity, containment, absolute composure. Nothing wild about it. There was a magnetism too, which I sensed beating in the rhythm of his infinite heart.

Zeus had been adopted into the exposed moorland farm where I was running a workshop with some of my dearest fellow practitioners. When the feral herd living on the nearby moors was reduced, he was one of the horses who were re-homed into captivity. His guardian, sensitive to his spirit, had allowed him to continue living as naturally as possible. Apart from the basic handling and domestication needed to care for him safely she wished to give him no 'training' at all.

That morning my co-practitioner and I had accompanied the five men and women to the field where Zeus and his grey field-mate Socks (short for Socrates) grazed. Once within the large round-pen in the centre of the rough grass expanse, with the horses on the outside of the enclosure in the field, we had formed a standing circle. After a short meditation we sat and shared, one at a time, our hopes and intentions for the journey we were undertaking that week.

Throughout the morning Zeus had remained at a distance from us, quietly nibbling around the perimeter of the field. Socks in contrast had brought an inquisitive playfulness and offered himself to every person who stepped out into his space. It had been a fruitful morning of insights and shifts in awareness.

An ageless wisdom

After the break a man called Axel took his turn. He had engaged fully in the morning process whilst also maintaining a sense of separateness. It was difficult to describe. He had not been aloof, in fact he had worked hard to reach out to us all. Yet a chilliness manifested from time to time when he seemed to slide discreetly back into himself. He was approaching retirement and had spoken earlier of wanting to find clarity during the week as to what his new direction should be. He was considering several options, including study, part-time contract work or taking a sabbatical to travel.

When Axel left the pen and entered the horses' area, the previously eager Socks distanced himself immediately. Within seconds he was at the other end of the field, filling his stomach. The man turned towards me, shrugging his shoulders in interrogation.

'Why has he done that?' As he spoke I felt a nuance of accusation and began to feel a little nauseous.

'Take a pause Axel, what is happening in your body right now? Can you describe what you are feeling?'

'I can't say as I feel anything, to be honest.' Then suddenly there was a barb in his voice. 'I am surprised that you allow this kind of thing to happen!'

I met the sharpness of his tone with softness in mine.

'What kind of thing Axel?'

'Horses refusing to work with us.'

I didn't respond. The irony of his statement was obvious given the willingness which Socks had shown for supporting the others throughout the morning.

'Ok – with *me*,' he conceded. 'For refusing to work with me. But I still think he should be better trained.'

This last phrase trailed away, the annoyance petered out, and I had a sense of a small boy in front of me, alone and unsure, not understanding the rules of his world. Yearning for help but not getting it.

Suddenly, as if he had materialised out of the mist Zeus stood like a statue a few strides from the pen. And that was when I felt it. This aura which opened onto the ages, this powerful, penetrating presence. He scrutinised Axel intently from behind the thick forelock over his eyes.

'Look over your shoulder, Axel.' I gestured.

He swivelled towards the motionless horse and I slid backwards so that the channel was open between them. I was disarmed by the intensity of the communication from Zeus to his student. The dampness in the air cast a cooling veil, blurring the horizon so that all receded around the man and horse.

'Can I go to him?' whispered Axel. I nodded.

For each careful step which Axel took towards Zeus, the pony took two backwards. Yet never losing eye contact. Like two dancers locked in the consuming steps of a tango they manoeuvred, until the man was sitting on a nearby fallen tree trunk, and the pony opposite him some twenty feet away. Zeus held the man securely with every ounce of his focus, then suddenly concluded the voiceless communion by dropping his head as if in a bow, swinging a shoulder round and walking to rejoin his field mate.

We came into our circle. There were no words to describe this non-verbal, inter-species exchange. Axel looked drained and as if the troubles of a lifetime had revisited him all at once.

Their rightful place

Two days later, it was Axel's turn again to have individual time with the horses. This time Zeus stayed much further from the man, yet still engaged him with the same intensity. They moved away from the group and held their own space out away from us all. The exchange ended with the same gracious bow.

'What can I say?' shrugged Axel when he returned to the group. 'That was something beyond anything I have experienced or even imagined was possible or can comprehend. All I know is that I received something I needed. Zeus, wow. When I needed him he came, just staring at me like that, with this understanding. It was like being cloaked in love. Like he knew everything about me ...'

The rest of us held the space respectfully, without comment. Axel looked down at the sandy soil, where his toe carved out a hollow.

'All my life I think I have been struggling with this deep-down loneliness. I've blamed other people when things get tough, heaped criticism on them and found fault to disguise how lost I feel. I've driven lots of people away by doing that. And I get so angry when they do, I lash out and then of course I lose them forever. Zeus saw through that. Stayed with me. I don't know what it all means, not yet, or if it will help me decide what to do with my life. But ...well ... maybe I don't need to decide. There was something about the way Zeus looked into my soul. That is what I need to learn to do, for myself. To see what he saw in there.'

Socks worked hard as we moved through the rest of the week, with Zeus offering exclusive access to Axel alone. When it was time to close our workshop we gathered in the centre of the round-pen in a circle. We all joined hands, leaving two gaps for the horses to join us energetically. But seconds after beginning the final meditation I peeked through closed eyelids to see both Zeus and Socks hovering by the gate. I signalled to

14

the group and discreetly slipped across to let them in. In the gaps that we had left Zeus and Socks positioned themselves quietly, taking their rightful place amongst us. After the ultimate words were uttered, Socks remained to claim as many caresses as he could while Zeus withdrew to the boundary of the farm. There I sensed his timeless aura cast its embrace towards the moor where the herd of his birth roamed: his sons, daughters, mares and rivals.

Having witnessed the power of Zeus' communication with Axel, I had no doubt that he was conversing with his own kind from afar. For a short time he had allowed us into his world, bestowed on us the magnificence of his spirit through which we had glimpsed timelessness. But his spirit remained forever with his kin running free across the high grounds. Over and beyond the fence his bond with them endured. I felt sad for him and all the creatures who have been kidnapped or reared into captivity, whilst knowing that realistically, it must now be thus. And he was one of the lucky ones, who had fallen upon a human home who respected his nature and let him be.

My thoughts turned to the horses and ponies for whom I was guardian. It no longer felt appropriate to call them 'mine'. I could not 'own' them. I was privileged to have them in my care and with that came a responsibility to provide as natural a lifestyle as possible.

4

Forgiving Our Sins

At the moment when Axel said that Socks lacked 'training' for his work, Zeus, the least 'trained' horse that I had ever worked with, offered himself willingly to support the man with his struggle. The irony didn't escape me and I found myself reflecting on this dynamic on the long journey home. It wasn't the first time that comments had been made about how well, or badly, horses had been prepared to teach human learners during the course of their encounters. The exchange I had witnessed between Zeus and Axel was the finest illustration that the ability of horses to help us heal has very little to do with any prerequisite skills instilled by their human guardians. That a horse, who was sprung from his natural habitat and obliged to adjust to our world, engages so generously with us, as Zeus had, is remarkable. This pony chose to help someone who had given him nothing.

Keepers of faith

I wondered, did the brown dappled pony see in Axel something of himself? The displacement, the anger, the confusion as to what the rules of the game were? How to respond to a situation of which he could not know the outcome, where all he could do was hold a patient and trusting heart? I imagined a human in the same circumstances. Taken from their family and held against their will, although treated kindly. How angry we would be, plotting to escape, struggling to adjust. Yet this horse and so many like him remain open to not only connect with but to help those who capture them. They keep faith.

A just transaction?

Many horses living amongst humans are not treated as well as Zeus. They are expected to deliver against a transaction to which they did not agree and may not understand. Sometimes they are hurt and punished when they ask for clarification or express an opinion. They tolerate the most nonsensical practices and unsatisfactory behaviour from their human keepers. And finally, when the unnatural lifestyle which we force upon them causes injury, or when they simply become too old to fulfil our aspirations, we discard them. Often they are killed, for convenience or for meat, or passed on as a problem to someone more naive. The horse is too often a commodity, an accessory, a toy or a cash machine. And still they forgive us our sins and make us better for our contact with them. Such is the horse.

Following the workshop with Zeus I continued swimming in his aura. I'd find my thoughts drifting to our encounter, my attention held as if he were right in front of me, there and then. I couldn't know that his inspiration would take me somewhere, sometime soon, that I would never have dared to go without him.

5

Lucy's Story

The clock is ticking

Lucy's olive skin stretched over her cheekbones like fine parchment. Her long lithe legs were clad in jeans and stylish country boots, whose recently-polished nut brown leather shone weakly through a veneer of moist mud.

'I'm not at all used to talking about myself,' she began. 'It's time I stopped bottling it all up though. A week's notice he gave me … I suppose I should be grateful for small mercies that he didn't jilt me at the altar. Anyway, that was a year ago and I'm seeing someone else now. But, well, things have got a bit rocky lately. He won't talk about the future, and I need to know where he stands … you know … whether he wants kids or not. The clock is ticking for me. I don't want to waste any more time on another commitment-phobe. I hoped that if I can learn how to communicate better with him, without getting so emotional about it, that could help. He might even come with me for a few sessions, who knows.'

The weight of expectation placed on this absent man weighed heavily.

'Tell me some more about your desire to have a family. What impact does this have on your life Lucy?' I asked.

As she talked in the still autumn air, a pattern unfolded of broken relationships. Her haste to secure a husband and father for her future children was often cited. The older she got the more urgent the matter became.

'I know I scare them off. But I would rather know sooner than later if they are not interested in kids. I am the wrong side of thirty-five now. I need to get on with it.'

The pressure to make things happen which Lucy exuded left no space to reflect, explore, even to breathe. It was best to go with the flow. 'Shall *we* get on with it then Lucy, and go to meet the horses?' I said, pulling my jacket around me and zipping it against the chill.

In the paddock Lucy instantly focused on Ruby, a chestnut mare whose beauty in that moment was even more irresistible than usual. Exquisite, fine, powerful yet soft, one of nature's jewels shining in the sunlight.

'I would like to groom her if that's OK?' Lucy asked. I nodded and she picked up a brush from the kit box on the ground. But as Lucy approached, Ruby darted to one side as if spooked.

'Can I use the halter please, to catch her. So I can groom?' Lucy asked straight away.

'Tell me about how that would help you,' I asked.

'Well I could make her stand still, then get on with the grooming. I'm sure she'd like it once we got going.'

'If she will allow you to put it on her then yes, that would be OK.'

Lucy returned brandishing the headgear but Ruby moved away even quicker than before.

'How do I make her come to me?' A frustrated tone was rising in her voice.

'She needs to trust you,' I coached. 'She has feelings of her own, it will take you time to understand what these are.'

'But how can I get to know her if she just keeps avoiding me?' Lucy was exasperated.

I left her question unanswered as it had not been addressed directly to me, but flung into the air somewhere nearby. Lucy paced and hovered around the wary mare for a few more moments before shouting in desperation: 'I just want her to come to me! Is it too much to ask?'

After a short pause I asked gently, 'Does anything about this situation feel familiar, Lucy?'

She looked at me and abruptly marched to the fence where she stared out towards the white horse chalked into the hill. Several minutes later a nudge on the back of the knee alerted her to the miniature cream-coloured Shetland pony who had snuck up behind. Lucy squealed with delight and soon Ellie's bottom lip was lolling with pleasure as she lovingly brushed the shaggy mane.

'I guess I got what I wanted in the end!' Lucy was laughing as she made her way back to me, Ellie trotting behind. 'That was so sweet. I love this creature!'

'I enjoyed witnessing you together Lucy. I am also curious about what originally caused you to walk away from me so suddenly. Before she came over, when you went over to the fence,' I asked.

'You asked if anything felt familiar. I guess you hit a nerve. The frustration of not being able to get to Ruby, of her stonewalling me, that felt just like it does with my boyfriend. When I try to engage him in conversations about the future he becomes unreachable. I know it's too early really to expect him to commit to me … but he could give me a clue about where he stands. Couldn't he?' Suddenly the anger was gone and doubt had taken its place. 'He says I am too pushy … the thing is, that is what my ex said too … so perhaps he is right. I just don't know how to be different.'

'And what was happening for you when Ellie approached?' I probed.

'I had this moment of honesty when I realised how I try to force relationships to be something they are not. Just like I was trying to make Ruby come to me and be brushed. If a horse, or a person, has wants of their own it is not for me to force them to do otherwise. I thought if Ruby doesn't want to be

20

groomed then I have to accept that. And that was when the pony came over. Ironically, it was when I stopped wanting to be with Ruby that Ellie gave me the closeness I crave.'

Lucy looked down to the ground, a little furtively, so I pushed a little more. 'Was there anything else you realised, in that moment of honesty?'

'Yes there is, although I hate to admit it. This guy I have been seeing ... I actually find him a bit boring ... but he fits the bill: decent, athletic, good job, has already had two kids with his previous wife. He would make a great dad, but if I am truthful there isn't the spark for me. Not like there should be. Not like there was with my ex.'

'That feels like an important detail Lucy!' I said with a smile. 'How might it be if you were to trust that somehow, somewhere, your integrity would attract the right person at the right time. Like it did with Ellie. That may or may not mean a family, for you ... of course ... because you won't have control over the time-line.'

'I could give it a try. Forcing the issue certainly isn't working. It would be difficult though because I want kids so badly. Do you understand that? Do you have children yourself?'

Do you have children?

Lucy had asked me that question, with no edge or intention, as casually as it is often posed, the question which for much of my life I had dreaded. That question which, if met with a 'no', can cut a conversation dead and leave loss, judgement, curiosity and pity hanging simultaneously in the air. That question which could take me back like lightning to a day in my twenties when I knelt on the patterned carpet of my mother's lounge with my newly born nephew gurgling on his back in front of me. When I knew that tug in the womb, that visceral longing. The desire proved stronger than reason and

21

later led me into a destructive marriage, which yielded no kids either.

'No, I do not have children,' I replied, taking care to breathe deeply.

'Oh.' Lucy looked uncomfortable. 'I'm sorry it was rude of me to ask … and intrusive.'

'Don't worry Lucy, I'm happy to share with you, if it helps,' I reassured her. 'I did want to have children. I can't know whether my experience was similar to yours, all I can say is that my life has yielded many other riches, that I could not have foreseen, in the absence of them. Undoubtedly it would have been very different if I had had a family. Whether I would have been more or less happy than I have been – I guess I will never know.'

Lucy looked pensive. 'I've been so focused on the one thing, I've forgotten that there is more than one route to happiness. A bit like I didn't notice the pony because I was so intent on Ruby. Maybe I'm missing opportunities by chasing the wrong men for the wrong reasons. Or scaring off the right men, for the right reasons, come to think of it!'

'Happiness is possible in all sorts of ways if we choose to have it Lucy. And there are lots of unhappy mothers as well as happy ones.'

'Yes, I guess you are right. It's just hard when everyone around you seems to be having children or is pregnant. I need to make some difficult decisions. But thank you.'

Lucy looked thoughtful but less troubled as she left. She went where I and thousands more women had gone before. Whatever the outcome was for her, I hoped that she would find love and fulfilment and shape the life she wanted with or without the experience of childbirth.

6

Horse Play

One too many

It is unusual for groups to be late arriving at the farm. A day in the countryside away from the workplace seems to inspire punctuality. Yet an hour after this workshop was due to start I was still waiting in the classroom with my team, the muffins drying out and the coffee past its best. My phone beeped. A text informed me that the board of directors of the household brand retailer who we were expecting had been delayed but that they had just left their hotel twenty miles away. I knew that probably meant one thing.

Two hours later than expected they began arriving, pale and tired. Some took a seat in the classroom and others disappeared back into their cars to take phone calls. My energy was now focused on managing my own frustration. By the time they were all present we had less than four hours to deliver something worthwhile.

Despite the excessive alcohol consumed and ensuing sleep deprivation, the team of fourteen men and one woman was buoyant. Voices boomed, jokes flew and making myself heard was difficult. Finally, I drew their attention long enough to start the introduction, but almost every time I paused for breath another round of verbal sparring would erupt. The rowdiness was like a forest fire – just when I thought it was extinguished a breeze would catch a spark and set it blazing again. I decided that I would let these flames burn themselves out. I stood quietly, bringing my awareness to my own body and my feet on the ground.

Banter or bullying?

I silently observed the chaos in the room. The dynamics amongst the group were thinly veiled as good-humoured banter. There were those who mocked and those who were mocked, those who made the jokes and those who were the butt of them. In simple terms there were those who bullied, and those who were belittled. It was shocking to be reminded of the organisational use of shame as a convenient tool of coercion which I had encountered at times during my own career.

The group was ignoring me, it was as if I wasn't there. The effort it was taking me to stay present told me I didn't really *want* to be there, either. Boundaries were being transgressed all around me, including my own. I noticed that I was feeling small then became aware of a tingling in my fingertips, a tightness in my jaw and fists. Behind the initial emotions a more dangerous one hovered – anger.

I looked out of the window and imagined bringing the tranquility which reigned out there into my being. I could see the horses with whom we would be working that day, and traced the sleek line of their shoulder and neck muscles with my eyes. They exuded the very embodiment of power. I tapped into it, let my anger go and imagined my energy growing beyond my 5'2" frame into that of a tall, broad horse, so big that it couldn't be contained by the classroom walls.

It didn't take long for the furore to abate and I seized the moment.

Tables turned

'We're going to go to meet the herd now,' I instructed. I knew I had little chance of effectively challenging this group regarding their behaviour in the next three hours. I would leave that to the horses.

Once in the fresh air I invited the group to disperse around the arena where, on the outside of the fence, they would be able to observe the horses interacting together in safety. Four geldings were set free in the large expanse of sand. Before too long William, a tiny caramel pony with thick jet-black mane and tail, set about stirring things up with the three full-size horses. Perhaps the most mischievous equine I have ever met, he quickly had the whole herd charging about the arena in a display of springtime fever. Their play was highly physical with the more dominant personalities vying for control. Even in the soft sand their hooves thundered, making dust fly as they reared, bucked, nipped and kicked.

The game reached its crescendo. William reared up and grabbed Oscar, a towering mass, by the throat. He spun round, reversed his huge hindquarters into the pony, bulldozing him to the opposite fence. Oscar did not hurt William – this was not an aggressive act. It was simply the sign from the herd alpha that playtime was over, that it had all got a bit out of hand. As all four horses stood there panting and snorting in relaxation, I observed the faces surrounding me and couldn't help smiling to myself. They were looking nervous to say the least.

Interpretation versus observation

We all gathered together on the lawn and I asked the group to share what they had observed about how the horses had behaved with each other. No-one said a word.

'What did you notice? Anything?' I asked again. Still silence. I prodded a little harder. 'We're going to be working with these horses now, loose in the field. How are you feeling about being amongst them, up close and personal?' It was my turn to be a little playful.

Someone spoke up from the back of the group. 'Are you sure that's going to be safe? They looked pretty violent and aggressive in there!'

'What led you to that conclusion?' I responded, keeping as neutral a tone as I could.

'I'd have thought it was obvious! They have just spent ten minutes kicking ten bells out of each other.' His tone suggested he thought me foolish for asking the question.

Now we were getting somewhere. 'What exactly did you see them doing? Tell me what you saw not what you think it meant.'

They became more animated now as they described the kicking, biting, running, chasing and charging.

'Great. So that was the physical behaviour. That is one thing. Second and more importantly is how you interpret that behaviour. What do you think it means? Any ideas?'

The consensus was that the horses had clearly been fighting, that they were dangerous and should not be approached by inexperienced humans.

'I am certainly not prepared to go anywhere near such vicious animals!' a voice rose from the ranks.

I acknowledged the comment with an 'I see' and continued. 'Let's take another look at what happened. Did you see any blood? Or any of the horses wanting to leave the arena, or running away to the corner to defend themselves with their tail between their legs? Or any one horse carrying out a sustained attack on any of the others until they were submissive and evasive?'

Voices murmured 'No' or heads shook in response to each of my questions.

'On the other hand, did you see each of the horses engaging willingly in the behaviour? And going back for more?'

'Errr. Yes.' Nods around the group backed up the affirmative statement of a man standing at the front.

'And what are the horses doing now?' I pointed to where two of the herd were now quietly standing side by side and the others were engaged in mutual grooming, dragging long teeth up and down each other's manes.

'Oh, I get it!' Someone called out. 'They were only playing!'

'Yes!' I said. 'Now you understand where the phrase horse play comes from. The play is sometimes rough, that's for sure. But it is aimed at establishing and maintaining the hierarchy and the dynamics of the herd as they are, as well as having fun.'

At the mention of the word 'fun' the group's unhelpful humour began to bubble up.

'Oy Rob, you need to be the first in! Test that animal magnetism of yours!'

'No! You go first. Show us what you're made of instead of dithering like you do with the unions.'

'OK guys, listen up!' I shouted. It was time to follow Oscar's example and turn my metaphorical hindquarters. Once all eyes were on me, I paused to give weight to what I would say next. 'Thank you for your attention. Does anything about the herd behaviour you've just witnessed feel similar to the dynamics in your own team?'

The truth will out

Silence fell, just for a moment. Then the woman, let's call her Jane, spoke up.

'Often in the boardroom we are very much like the horses were. We rarely take each other seriously; the jokes are usually at someone else's expense. And well, we are just very loud and bawdy on the whole. And if that is how I feel, I dread to think

27

what the rest of our organisation thinks. What you all claim to be banter could appear at best rude, at worst aggressive.'

Jane's intervention met with passive assent and as we divided to work in smaller numbers the conversation turned to hopes for a new way of operating. We moved through the rest of the day and I didn't worry that most of it was spent either having lunch or tea and cake. The important work had already been done. What needed to be said had been said and I hoped, perhaps optimistically, that for the sake of the thousands of their employees this team would find a way of being together more constructively.

It was the only group I have ever worked with who I was glad to see leave when the clock struck five. Yet this had been another magical lesson for me through which I felt a magnetic partnership with the horses. By relying on them to do their work, by inviting them into the learning space as expert teacher, bowing to their intuition and extraordinary clarity, I had been supported, even looked after. When I didn't know what to do next, once again, they had been there with the answer.

Playing out in front of me I had that day been reminded of how readily the shaming of others can be used as a means of control. And how, if you are on the receiving end, your self-belief shrivels whilst a destructive rage simmers inside. I had lived this cycle more than once in my adult life. Horses had held my hand during the long climb back to self-worthiness, seeing in me that which I had lost sight of myself.

7

Choosing Happiness

I had an early mentor on the subject of happiness – my grandmother. It was strange because she had every reason not to be happy. Yet I remember her as one of the most serene people I have ever known.

Lilian, or Lil as she was known, had developed rheumatoid arthritis at the age of 40. It was wartime Britain and she, my grandfather, aunt and mother lived in one of the terraced dock-workers' houses in inner-city Liverpool. They were poor. The girls had two dresses each, made by my grandmother. Zips were beyond their means so Lil would every morning take the same piece of thread and sew the back of her daughters' dresses closed, undoing the stitches at bedtime. Food and medication were scarce and in their cold damp house condensation ran permanently down the inside of the windows. My mother used to tell me how as a child she was always cold and hungry. Lil's rheumatoid arthritis quickly took hold bringing pain, disability and still more poverty with it. My grandfather turned to drink and gambling, I was told, and the family lived off my mother's wages when she went out to work as a typist at the age of 14.

Lil's disease progressed, then in 1949 came a breakthrough in medical science. A new wonder-drug, cortisone, became widely used in the treatment of anti-inflammatory disease. Lil was one of the thousands of patients liberally prescribed this medicine. It appeared to stop pain and halt arthritic disease. Pharmaceutical giants and doctors alike claimed that it would even give the body the chance to generate new cells. Before the devastating side-effects of the drug were publicly known (skin and bone destruction) my grandmother's spinal column had collapsed and her skin resembled tissue paper which split open into sores and ulcers. She was sent to my parents' house from hospital to die, her head held up by a rigid leather collar and her body crumpled like a bag of bones in the chair. I was two years old.

Die Lilian did not, but suffer she did. Yet a smile was always available for us as we grew up. A formless, paralysed hand would rest on my hair as I sat at her feet and I remember the delicate fragility of her skin as I stroked her jelly-like fingers. My brothers and I would revolve around her chair from which she was lifted periodically to lie on the bed by my mother or grandfather. Like three fledgling swallows we would chatter, begging for a story (she was a superlative orator), showing her our drawings or reading to her when we were old enough. On sunny days and before he also succumbed to arthritis, my grandfather Charlie would push her in her wheelchair to the park, with us tripping alongside. She endured agony all those years but rarely showed it.

As I grew older, and brought to her my inconsequential troubles, her counsel was gently offered. 'The thing is Pammie, you must never take things for granted. Not even walking or running. Enjoy the life you have. Now go and have a wash and buck yourself up. That'll make you feel better.'

And strangely enough, it usually did.

Lilian passed away at the age of 73, 13 years after she had been sent home to die.

Grateful. And yet...

My grandmother's words accompanied me as I settled into Wiltshire. I cherished the friendships developing and the beautiful countryside which opened from my doorstep. I'd take

30

the dogs walking along the nearby tow path where the kingfisher would fly its electric blue trace and the gliding swans presented my own private ballet. The field where my herd now dwelt under the eye of the great chalk horse became a haven and a base for long rides out with Ruby. I loved it all. The collaboration I was developing with the farm where I based my client programmes was blossoming and business was thriving with the support of a world-class team of colleagues. What more could I want?

And yet … there was still this part of me which wasn't satisfied. In Lilian's lifetime 'Gratitude' had not yet become formulated into a popular strategy for self-improvement. It was simply how my grandmother got through each painful hour and every repetitive day. Appreciative and positive awareness of the love which was available to her made the unbearable bearable and allowed positive energy into a place where resentment or bitterness may have dwelt. In spite of this early learning, and the professional knowledge I had acquired about the benefits of practising thankfulness, still my spirit was restless.

I was discovering that choosing happiness wasn't just about counting my blessings. The quiet but insistent voice of dissatisfaction was challenging me to do something different. Could I learn to distinguish which yearnings were born from my soul and would carry me all the way to my destiny, from those which come forth from a place of insecurity or ego-driven ambition?

My internal critic took me to task. Why couldn't I be content with this lifestyle which was so good? An echo of a voice from long ago scolded – it sounded like my mother's – I was so ungrateful.

8

My Book

Spring 2014

'You should write a book,' he said.

At the end of the two-hour Skype call this wasn't what I expected to hear from the branding consultant I had hired to revamp my website. Kindly and skilfully he had turned me inside out during the interview on all aspects of my work.

'Yeah! Right!' I didn't take his comment seriously, and tried to move the conversation back to the project in hand.

'I'm serious,' he insisted. 'How you came to discover the healing capacity of horses, and what that has led to. There is a great story in there. Important for your brand, too.'

I dismissed the notion out of hand, but a seed was lodged. It just rested, in my psyche, digging itself in and slowly taking root. Me? Write a book! I would chuckle to myself every now and again. How amusing.

And yet ... I enjoyed writing short blogs for my newsletter and website. People liked them. I'd loved writing essays at school. Maybe, just maybe ... What if I tried? What might it be to attempt something so big, which I thought impossible? I could do it, just for me, no-one need ever read it ... or even know.

So, little by little my book came into being, long before I put pen to paper. Until one day, as the summer holidays began and my client workload diminished I typed at the top of the screen: 'My Story'.

Often I wrote through the blurred vision created by my tears. As I walked back through my adult life, the older, wiser woman holding the hand of her junior, I realised that there was still some emotional tidying up to do. I cried for the fifteen-year-old whose father had left, the hopeful bride-to-be whose lover moved on, for the bereaved daughter, friend, step-mother and sister, the downtrodden wife and the lost young woman who had rediscovered herself several times over.

I laughed too, almost as much, and celebrated as I revisited my triumphs. I connected with all the goodness past and present. As my fingers clattered across the keyboard it was as if all those I had lost sat with me in my small office overlooking the golden wheat-fields of summer. Until I came to write about January 2012. Then a darkness descended and I clicked the document shut. Filed it away. It was too soon. Too raw.

The shadow of trauma

I watched him die, after all. In a matter of hours and days. The disease disguised as influenza was diagnosed too late as the stealthy killer sepsis, which takes more lives than cancer each year. My brother's body and all its defences were quickly overwhelmed. Two years later my professional training told me that not only was I still grieving but that I was also traumatised.

So although something new in me had been awakened through writing, I knew I could go no further. I wasn't strong enough to face what had happened in this particular chapter. My book was put away. It had been a stupid idea in the first place.

33

9

Ellie

Pocket-sized ponies

Ellie came as one of a pair. Two almost identical miniature Shetland ponies – sisters, or mother and daughter, without a doubt. Distinguishable only by a nuance of hue in their 'café-au-lait' coats and the different lengths of their extravagant, cream manes and tails. The darker fur on Ellie's nose formed the shape of a heart around her fuzzy nostrils. Dawn had slighter shorter hair and a wider, more square face. For strangers it was hard to know which was which unless they were standing side by side.

The ponies had belonged to a previous partner. Originally purchased for his young children they had become full-time lawn mowers on his two-acre property when his ex-wife left taking the kids with her. Obese, with toes like Aladdin's slippers, dental problems and infested with lice, Dawn and Ellie had become semi-feral. Within weeks of my meeting this man the Shetlands became my project. I won their confidence and nursed them back to health. There was no question of me leaving them behind when he and I went our separate ways.

With my two horses Winston and Ruby, the Shetlands formed the herd who would support me with much of the equine assisted learning and therapy I offered in Wiltshire. Larger programmes for the corporate sector would take place at the farm with which I was collaborating, where there were better facilities and a herd of fifteen available to join us. But my gang would work with longer term clients and smaller groups.

Although similar in appearance the ponies' personalities were starkly different and there was nothing diminutive about either of them. Dawn was calm, independent and confident, with astute problem-solving skills and a tenacity for breaking out through fencing. Ellie was nervous and wary of unknown adults, unless she was drawn to work with them, in which case she would make herself known most persistently.

Children's friend

Ellie adored young children, the smaller the better, towards whom she would magnetise from a distance. She'd walk beside them, taking care to slow down so they could keep up and to allow them space when squeezing through gates. Young arms wrapped around her neck, button noses buried in the mattress of a mane, hands tugging at her tail as they brushed: she received all with love, tolerance and gentleness of spirit.

Perhaps the most vocal pony I have ever known, Ellie communicated with a fanfare. As our relationship developed, she would respond to my calls with high pitched whinnying. She aspired to be the lead mare and vied with Ruby, four times her size, for this coveted position. The Shetland's weaponry: piercing squeals, a whipping with her immense tail and, revoltingly, a willingness to cover herself in steaming, fresh dung. Although she rarely stood up to the flattened ears of her rival, she succeeded in becoming the almost constant companion of the alpha gelding in the herd, Winston, to whom she became devoted. Their closeness was endearing. His bulk would tower over her as they grazed in tandem around the field, she trailing him like a baby elephant in the wake of its mother. In heavy wind and rain, he would tenderly shelter her from the elements with his broad neck and shoulders. Her life-long bond with Dawn still remained intact and it was for

35

resting and sleeping that they would come together, side by fluffy side, their heads lolling in unison as they dozed.

The impact of this small pony on the youngsters who worked and played with her was something really special. She would touch them with both her hearts: the one on her nose and the one which radiated understanding and healing from within. She helped a number of traumatised children of all ages to find their voice and their confidence.

For adults Ellie's presence could be equally life-changing. She had this way of singling out particular individuals whose attention was invariably directed towards the bigger horses. They would suddenly feel a polite little nudge in the crook of their knee and there she would be, inviting contact. She helped people to soften into self-compassion and pave the way for change when grappling with issues from bereavement to career crisis. Where matters of parenthood – actual or unfulfilled – were unresolved she would invariably volunteer her wisdom and calming presence.

Beside the snowdrops

Ellie, who brought me so much joy, and touched the lives of all those she encountered, passed away swiftly of natural causes one sunny February afternoon. She chose a moment when I was just feet away from her enjoying the sight of her basking in the winter warmth. She swayed, staggered, then toppled. It was over in a matter of seconds. In the copse beyond, an abundance of snowdrops peeped through the russet carpet of fallen autumn leaves.

As I had with my brother and mother at the moment that they passed, I had a sense of Ellie all around me. A presence without form, yet with all the qualities which she had possessed in life. I wondered at how such a small pony could fill this large field, but she did. I plaited flowers into her mane, cradling her pretty head in my lap, giving thanks that she had passed so peacefully and that I had had the privilege to share the moment with her. How fortunate I had been to have the joy of caring for this sweet, kind, wise, creature in her final years.

I noticed after a while that I was shivering, perhaps from shock, as much as the cold. Soon it would be dark and I had to leave her and go home to make the necessary practical arrangements. But first the herd had to say their goodbyes too. By chance I had left them enclosed in the corral while Ellie had been finishing her feed. She barely had any teeth left and it took her much longer to eat than the others. When I opened the slip rails they trotted over to Ellie's body, circled her then stopped abruptly in a line.

The herd's tribute

Ruby, the lead mare of the herd, was the first to approach. She touched Ellie gently with her nose, walked away, then returned to explore again, several times over. It was as if she was seeking understanding. Then, as her head dropped down to the pony she threw her head up with a spine-chilling, high pitched screech, repeated again and again, simultaneously kicking out violently with her hind leg. She moved away and the other two came one after the other to sniff the lifeless muzzle. Dawn shook herself from head to tail creating a cloud of dust around her and whinnied loudly. Winston simply touched her gently and turned to face away. Dawn and Ruby took up positions near him also with their backs to the dead pony. Motionless, they all stood sentry as if protecting her as she slept. Or perhaps, as she passed.

A unique consciousness

I have tried to give a factual rather than anthropomorphic account of what happened. What was clear, however, after witnessing the herd's response to Ellie's death was that horses (and other animals) possess a consciousness and powerful emotions which are uniquely their own.

It is sometimes said that equines teach us by mirroring our emotions back to us. This term diminishes the horses as well as the adventure which *we* have into the self-revelation which can surround our interactions with them. They do not blandly reflect the moods and behaviour of those humans around them. Far from it – they have their own emotional experience in relation to us. It is by our mindful observation and awareness of what they express that we gain insights which help us to be better at being who we are.

Just a mirror?

To talk of horses mirroring our emotions is to deny them their validity and to deprive ourselves of potentially transformational experience. When we learn with horses, they are not our tool. We are entering into a unique, vibrant, many-layered dynamic, which is the manifestation of all that is wondrous about the natural world itself.

And if we can lapse into seeing horses as reflections of ourselves, do we also fall into the same trap with other humans? Is this why we fail to understand 'the other', because we are expecting them to be like us? And when they don't meet our expectations we judge, dismiss, become frustrated, try to bend them to our will, or question our own self-worth?

Might it be that learning to honour and communicate with another species helps us to reframe the way that we perceive each other, as well as how we might see ourselves? For whether we are projecting our inadequacies onto others, or protecting ourselves with façade, horses will always see us for who we are, and call us to be who we are meant to be.

Being with what is

On Ellie's passing and in the days of shared transition which followed I felt that I became connected with my herd in a new way. Bereavement had always been my domain – my mother, father, brother and stepfather. I had been able to witness the impact of *my* emotions and how I managed them, on the horses. They had helped me to heal, guiding me to own my feelings, releasing my anxieties and shedding the tears I needed to.

Now our loss was shared, yet our experience was also different. For me there was shock, sadness, guilt (could I have done more to care for my pony?) and worry (would the others be alright without her?). The horses, they looked for their friend and I could see too that their relationships with each other were reconfiguring. But there was no drama, no recrimination, no 'if-only's' or 'I should have done's'. They were simply at peace with what was.

And that perhaps, is the essence of the horse's gift to us. How to be, with whatever is. As I said goodbye to Ellie I acknowledged that, as far as grieving my brother was concerned, I still had some way to go. Losing her also gave me cause to reflect on what it meant to be separated from my herd by the mile which lay between my home and theirs, where access was difficult and there was no power or lighting.

In earnest I began to look for a new location for the horses. The nearest place was a half hour's drive away. That would not do either. I resigned myself to leaving them where they were. But I would find myself logging on to browse websites advertising equestrian properties for rent or sale with increasing regularity. The call of my promise was becoming louder.

10

Josephine's Story

She walked into the room bringing a touch of nature with her. There was something undefinably mystical about this woman that I was meeting for the first time. I felt as if the thick hair which bounced on her shoulders should have been plaited with ivy and daisy heads. The smart, ironed clothes and efficient notebook she carried were incongruent.

'Hi. I'm Josephine.' She rammed the tense fingers of her right hand into my outstretched palm. 'I'm here because I'm stuck. Fed up. Not sleeping. So annoyed with myself for feeling like this, it's not like me at all. And it's really pathetic, I have no right to be down.'

Josephine's speech was delivered as if she was in a real hurry to get to the end of it. I was about to open my mouth in reply when she added, 'Oh and also I came here because I am terrified of horses. But my daughter loves them and wants me to take her for riding lessons when she is old enough.' She rolled her eyes. 'I desperately want to make this happen, reckon I have about two years to get over my nerves.'

A perfect life

Josephine worked for a local financial services company. Her husband had a job at the same organisation and she described a comfortable existence.

'My marriage? Yes, it's good. Frank was my school sweetheart, we are like two peas in a pod. He still leaves me cheeky little notes in my lunch box when I'm not looking. The kids are great, my older son doing well at junior school and the little one, well, she is just a treasure. She is six now. Although I would be happier if she wasn't so mad on ponies!' Josephine chattered breathlessly of the certainty which plagued her that her daughter would get hurt if she went riding. Until she suddenly slammed her hands flat on her thighs, 'On and on I go! Sorry, I am so wasting your time.'

'Whatever you bring here is welcome Josephine, really. Tell me a bit more about being fed up, what is it like?'

'Oh, I just get ratty. I nitpick over little things in the house, the mess the kids make, the fact that Frank has left his soggy bath towel on the floor. I find it hard to do spontaneous things too, like I used to, everything has to be scheduled otherwise I get panicky. I suppose with the house to run and job to do, it's no wonder. I don't have much time to relax.'

'And tell me about your fear of horses.'

'I badgered my parents for riding lessons when I was little, I was a nightmare. Just like my little girl Phoebe. Then the first time I went I fell off and broke my wrist. My mum went crazy. That was more scary than the horse throwing me! I never went again, she kept on at me that I would probably get an even worse injury. I don't want to stifle Phoebe in the same way. Having said that I can't sleep some nights for obsessing about her having an accident.'

'If this is keeping you awake, I think we had better start with the horses. Then come to the fed-up bit afterwards? How does that sound?'

Fill the gap with fact not catastrophe

Outside a gale was brewing and the sky threatened rain. Across the fence from us grazed Molly and Polo, two gentle, older mares. As I led Josephine into a short relaxation exercise they drifted closer until their noses were resting on the pine rail in front of us.

'As you prepare to open your eyes Josephine, be mindful to carry on breathing when you do so, and keep feeling your feet on the ground.'

'Oh! I wasn't expecting that!' Josephine was delighted when she saw them. 'They are so close, so huge! And I am not even worried.'

Before the end of the session the wild-haired woman was grooming Polo in her stable. The heavens had opened and it seemed the most sensible place to be. Even these close confines didn't unnerve Josephine as she struck up a rapport with her equine partner. She passed the brush down the horse's body rhythmically, each stroke slower than the last, each touch more potent. Polo began to snooze and my own eyelids became heavy in the comforting space. There is something about being in the vicinity of a relaxed horse which calms the spirit and slows the beat of the heart.

'I can't believe I am doing this, I really can't. I thought it would take weeks for me to even touch a horse.' Josephine's wonder sparkled like that of a child opening an unexpected gift on Christmas Day. 'Are you sure she is OK with what I am doing?'

'Yes I am sure,' I replied. 'See how her bottom lip is wobbling? And the muscle-tone is soft in her neck, with her head lower than her withers – that's the bit here at the base of her neck – and her eyelids are closing. That is how you know she is calm. If you can learn how to read the emotions of a horse it is so much easier to stay safe as well as give them what they need. Perhaps if you learn some more about horses that will put you in a good place to support your daughter when she makes a start?'

'Yes, you're right. I feel so much safer just knowing that Polo likes me being here.'

'Sometimes when we are afraid of something it can be just because we lack information. The problem comes when we fill in the gaps with catastrophe.'

'Yes and I am a master at that! At night my imagination has been inventing all kinds of horrors based on nothing other than my fear.'

The boxes we build

The next session came a month later. Josephine reported sleeping better and was excited about meeting Polo again.

'And how about the fed-up bit? How is that going, because we didn't have time to explore that last time?'

'Funnily enough I haven't noticed it so much. I have been much more relaxed and tolerant of everyone. Surprisingly what has been more on my mind is excitement at seeing Polo again. It was such a lovely experience. I can't believe I have deprived myself of horses all these years because of a belief which my mother put in my head. Because of a story I have told myself.'

There was a vitality to these phrases which drew me back to them later in the session. We were sitting in the field, observing the herd in silence as they moved around. Josephine suddenly sighed deeply, as if she had been holding her breath for years. This was my cue.

'You mentioned earlier that you have denied yourself the pleasure of horses, Josephine. That felt important. Tell me, what else might you have held yourself back from?'

I could tell she was struggling to form the words as she stared into the middle-distance. 'I love my family, so much. But sometimes I feel as if I have built myself a box and thrown away the key.'

'And what are the stories which keep you in the box?' I asked.

'That I have to be a good mum and wife, or Frank won't love me. That I have to stay in my job because we need the money. That if I am away from home even just for one night something bad will happen to the kids. That if I let them do risky things they will get hurt. Everything just feels – well, so precarious. Keeping control of everything is difficult.'

'What are you afraid of, Josephine?'

Behind her blank expression something was crystallising and I signalled for her to carry on grooming Polo.

The soft brush stayed in Josephine's pocket and she used her right palm to stroke the patchwork fur. Polo stayed within reach of the hand which had started to instinctively scratch one of her itchy spots.

Without warning Josephine briskly withdrew. 'OK we're done here! She has had enough.'

I sensed that the lid of the box was closed with Josephine firmly back inside.

Never too late

'We have ten minutes left,' I coaxed. 'Why don't you enjoy the sunshine with Polo for a little longer.'

Without comment the woman sat beside the pony, stock still, as if in a trance. In a little while Polo suddenly began to yawn, and lick her lips, she was relaxing. Something had shifted. I drifted over and sat next to the upright human form.

'How are you doing?'

'Better, much better. Thank you.' Josephine said as she looked up at me.

'And what just happened?'

'I acknowledged what it meant to have given up on the aspirations I had before marrying. I feel guilty because I wouldn't be without the family, in any way. How could I possibly? But there were other hopes and dreams I put aside. I suppose that makes me sad still. And now, I don't know, it's like I need the life I chose to be perfect. Because if it isn't then

44

I gave up the other things for nothing. So I have to control everything. Nothing can go wrong. It is utterly exhausting.'

'Perhaps there is another option, Josephine? To reach out *now* for your ambitions. What was it that you really wanted to do, back then when you were 18?'

'You are going to think I am mad. I wanted to make rocking horses. I was very good at woodwork. And obsessed with horses of course. I made one in the sixth form for my assessed project. But who would be crazy enough to try doing that for a living?'

'Perhaps you might be?' I smiled. 'By acquiring new information this afternoon you achieved what you have been hankering after – to be close to a horse. I wonder what would happen if you looked into how your business idea might be possible? You know about both finance and woodwork. You have the skills you need to succeed.'

Congruence brings creativity

During the following months Josephine and I continued to meet. Downtime with Polo and an increasing confidence around the herd helped Josephine to rediscover a creative energy. She developed a plan for a small enterprise making and selling rocking horses. She and her husband had a large garage which they converted into a workshop and she sourced enough second-hand tools and machines to make a start. At our final meeting, before I had time to welcome her, she slapped a sheaf of papers on the table.

'Ta-da! There it is! The business plan. All agreed by the bank. I can make this work!'

I contrasted how Josephine now looked to the first occasion we met. There was no crease ironed into her jeans, no clipboard or polished nails. Her outer appearance was congruent with the creative, earthy energy of her physical presence. I mused if she would call her first rocking horse Polo.

45

In Josephine I had witnessed an undoing of the knots she had tied around herself, which in turn gave birth to an eruption of ideas and enthusiasm. The love for her family which she had previously verbalised, was no longer bound in language of duty and sacrifice. It sung its melody in every cell of her body. She had given herself permission to imagine something else could be possible and had dispelled much of her uncertainty by practical fact-finding, leading to the transformation of a fantasy into a grounded plan. I had seen that she needed to do this. It struck me like a bolt that I had to do this myself.

11

The Body's Journey

My colleagues will tell you that on the morning of a programme I always forget to take something with me however many lists I have written. This morning was no different. I realised that my sunscreen was still sitting on the kitchen table as I reversed down my driveway. It was going to be hot, I would fry without it. Leaving the engine running I slipped back into the house. That is when the first sweat came. By the time I had stepped into the hallway, my freshly laundered white shirt was soaked with perspiration. I could feel the unpleasant damp patches under my arms trickling their way around my body. Even my shins seemed to be oozing. Looking frantically at my watch, I calculated that I had enough time to get changed. I grabbed three shirts from the wardrobe, put one on and then draped two in the car should I need to freshen up later. I knew what this was. I wasn't ill, I was menopausal. It seemed that not only was there an emotional, professional and spiritual change process afoot, but a physiological one too.

I was spared mood swings and low energy levels but I despaired at the inability of my body to regulate its temperature. Treasured items of clothing (the warm ones) now stayed in the wardrobe, cooling bamboo bedding was purchased and dietary advice followed. Tactics were everything. Never sit near the radiator at a pub or restaurant, get a seat by the door or window. Always wear layers of clothes, ideally natural fabrics. Cut down on 'heating' food and drinks – spicy dishes, chilli, tea, coffee and alcohol. Drink lots of cold water. Taking plenty of exercise was not a problem, with two energetic terriers and three equines to look after. I was also fortunate to work from home so could wear what was comfortable, which was sometimes very little at all.

It was inescapable. From the benign to the difficult, the changes of menopause were imposing themselves forcefully. As my herd had guided me at Ellie's passing, I had to learn, as far as my body was concerned, to be with what was. To care for my physical self during the process, it seemed that self-love, self-care and gentleness were more needed than ever.

The liberation of age

In a strange way this womanly transition was liberating. I was released from the tyranny which my hormonal balance had wielded during my adult life, causing monthly discomfort and emotional ups and downs. I had finally passed the point, too, when I could have conceived any children. Whilst I had long since embraced the fact that I would not have kids mentally and emotionally, that my body had caught up helped to free me of any latent longing. Energy was released and strangely it began to feel as if the older I got, the nearer I felt to the girl of twenty who walked barefoot one Sunday morning on a deserted Biarritz beach.

12

France Discovered

Pau 1982-83

The coach pulled into Biarritz coach terminus, near the seafront, at around 6am. The sumptuous hotels, casinos and villas, shining white, cream and gold along the shoreline, were still sleeping. I wheeled my huge suitcase down to the paved walkway which ran at the head of the beach. I took off my socks and walked across the golden expanse to paddle in the quietly rippling, tepid waves. After spending 24 hours travelling it was bliss for my swollen feet. I was alone in this foreign country, on my way to study French at the University of Pau for the year. No mobile phone in those days, not even any accommodation arranged at my destination or someone waiting to meet me. I don't remember being afraid, only elated, to have this episode unfolding mysteriously before me.

Later I bought my first ever croissants, I couldn't quite believe how delicious they were, then boarded a train to Pau where I would be living for the next ten months. I arrived at around noon, the high sun igniting the bougainvillea blooms all around me. There was a quaint cable car to transport travellers from the valley in which the railway line sat, up a steep, deep embankment to the plateau where the town, once a playground for Victorian royals, spread its nobility. Dragging my large suitcase behind me, I tumbled out of the tiny carriage onto a leafy square shaded by colossal plane trees.

What now? Being lunchtime and a Sunday in France, there was no-one around to ask for directions. For the first time I felt unnerved. I was weary and my belongings weighed four times as much as they did when I packed them. Then into my view came an elderly man on a creaking bicycle. He stopped beside me. Behind a moustache which could have been mistaken for the tail of a Persian cat, his wrinkled face was kind. He was wearing a beret and had a baguette wrapped in tissue paper strapped to his back. I could hardly believe my eyes. When he enquired, I explained my situation.

'Come, come!' he boomed. 'My sisters run a guest house, they will have a room for you.'

Parking his bike against one of the trees the monsieur gallantly took my case. Several blocks away we arrived at an old-fashioned hotel with fine lace draped in the tall windows. I was ushered through the hallway and its jungle of dusty rubber plants to a dining room where I was fed Sunday lunch. For a small fee the two gentrified ladies lodged me until I found a student flat to share some two weeks later. Thus was cemented my love for this host country, begun in my early teens when I had visited a French pen-friend and her family.

Fontainebleau 1985-87

After graduating I secured an administrative job at a business school an hour south of Paris. I didn't really care what I did, as long as it was in France. Working differed from the carefree existence I had enjoyed as a student but nonetheless this country suited me. Each day brought new lessons and delightful rewards. Even the most mundane of office tasks taught me some new piece of vocabulary and engaged me in putting the language skills I had learned at university to use. Every trip to the market on a Saturday morning introduced me to a new kind of vegetable, fruit, cheese or fish which I would prepare following the culinary advice given by the produce

50

vendors. The diversity and freshness of the food available captivated me, as did the fine cuisine and the sophistication of the average Frenchwoman's wardrobe. I had my hair cut in the closely cropped 'gamine' style and worked hard to emulate them but suspect that I never quite managed it.

The French protected leisure and family time. They took all their holidays, had proper lunch hours and rarely worked at the weekend. Value was placed on the natural environment of which they were proud, walking, picnicking and making use of the beauty spots which surrounded them. Expertise in growing vegetables, foraging mushrooms in the forest or seafood at the coast was not unusual. I quickly grew to admire and enjoy this culture I found. When, after two years, I returned to the UK to advance my career it was only meant to be for a short while. I was not to know that almost thirty years would pass before I would set foot on French soil once again.

13

The Return

Linda – June 2015

The cliff-top restaurant was so close to the edge that it felt like we might drop into the water beneath. The turquoise spangled sea undulated hypnotically to the horizon, the cry of gulls piercing the air even above the noises of the restaurant. Almost thirty years since I had left France in my mid-twenties, I was back. The clatter of plates, chink of glass, pouring of wine, scraping of cutlery on plates, waiters efficiently darting between tables and the rise and fall of merry conversation. This place was a feast for the ears, eyes, nose and palate. I loved hearing the French language spoken around me. I was transported on the collective energy of shared companionship, of loved ones coming together to break bread. It was an energy of appreciation which pulsed in this busy, basic seaside restaurant. And, of course, the food – that was mouth-watering.

After lunch we had our photograph taken sitting shoulder to shoulder on the stone wall of the terrace. Three women, friends and former colleagues, all of a certain age, with shared histories. Only two of us would meet again in health.

Later on, Linda sat on the promenade with her daughter while Sarah and I rolled up our trousers and walked across the sand flats. The tide was going out fast, depositing great mounds of seaweed to navigate. Returning breathless, with salt-caked legs and skin alive with the charge in the air, I felt like a girl again.

Linda was convalescing with her daughter and family following surgery to reduce a brain tumour. An indomitable and robust woman who swept through life like a colourful wave, she courageously made plans for future travel, education and exciting work projects. We treasured every moment together, eeking it out, making it count. I soaked up her electric smile and stored it. Rendered frail by her illness, she needed to rest and after two unforgettable days together the three of us hugged goodbye.

Mayenne

It was a holiday of two halves. From Brittany I travelled to Mayenne to visit some more friends who had relocated there some two years earlier. They had sold up in England so that they were in a position to buy land for their horses. Unlike me, they didn't speak French. In contrast to the pathos of my time with Linda, the next few days flowed lightly. From a family holding together under tragic circumstances to a couple for whom a new life was beginning.

Their home could not have been more idyllic. Rambling roses in the garden, hedgerows loaded with Spring flowers and herbs, the horses living beyond a small kidney shaped lake which glinted beside the orchard. Wildlife making its presence felt and the most glorious of weather. I was guided round the local beauty spots and riverside walks.

My forays into equestrian real estate websites had taken me, remotely, to France. Land was more affordable than in the United Kingdom. But emigrate here on my own? Could I really contemplate such a move? Would I ever see anyone if I lived alone so deep in the countryside? It seemed like it could be a very lonely existence. And although part of me craved what my friends were creating, all I could think of was the long dark evenings swallowing me up.

On the last night of my stay we had reserved a table at a small cafe in one of France's 'petites cités de caractère'. The mediaeval village with pilgrim's chapel, enigmatic water meadows, curling river and hilltop views has drawn artists and visitors throughout the centuries. On arrival we were greeted by the patron, an attractive man with what my friend called 'come to bed eyes' and 'been to bed hair', who explained that due to a mains water leak the kitchen was regrettably closed. He had taken the liberty, however, of booking us into another establishment for our meal, but hoped we would stay for a complimentary aperitif on his terrace before we went.

As we sipped our drinks three large vans, blazoned with the county's water company logo, pulled up on the mediaeval bridge adjacent to us, completely blocking the narrow road. Eight workers in fluorescent jackets spilled out and started dragging large coils of tubing from the vehicles. The patron spoke with one of them and the whole troop swooped onto the terrace in a wave of bonhomie. Bottles of beer and sparkling wine were handed around, workwear was draped on the back of chairs and the party began. Their voices echoed through the town, oblivious to the traffic which was being forced to find a detour, well into the late evening.

Our meal was served in the garden of the restaurant to which we had been diverted. When I went inside, I discovered that the walls were adorned with dozens of paintings, mostly of horses. It transpired that our hostess was an artist who painted all winter and cooked for tourists all summer. One image drew me close. A horse's head appearing as if from a dark mist, with deep, soft eyes.

'That is my forever horse,' the Dutch woman smiled at the canvas before me. 'He is gone now, but he is the one who changed my life. Whose spirit lives on within me.'

I asked if she had used a photograph or sketches when she created the picture, because it was so real. 'Ah, no,' she replied. 'I see every detail of him, every day, I just need to close my eyes and he is there.'

The next day I went back to buy the picture before returning to the UK. It felt important.

Sarah and I saw Linda again, a few months later when she returned to the UK for hospice care. The following winter we planted crocuses on her grave. How abruptly our destiny changes and our opportunity for this life can end.

14

Jim's Story

'It isn't just the missing of my wife which I struggle with, it's that she was the only person who ever really saw me for who I am. With her, I didn't have to be better than I am, or different. I could just be me. There was this easy acceptance I never had in my first marriage.' Jim told me how his office romance with his late wife had blossomed after parallel divorces.

Best mates

'It's funny, there wasn't that much spark at first. Aileen was like one of the lads really, and she wouldn't have minded me saying that either. She was the only woman I've ever met who didn't baulk at getting her leathers on and riding pillion on my motorbike. She had some guts. God she did …' His mind went somewhere else. Briskly he pulled down his sweater, smoothed the creases and sat up straight.

'I never really felt like I fitted in anywhere, you know, I'm not sure why. Not until I met Aileen. Then I stopped caring what other people thought. And how we used to laugh! I'd have done anything for her, you know. If only I could have swapped places. Now I'm lost.'

I could see that he really was.

'And how do you feel that coming here to spend time with us will help?' I asked.

'Someone recommended you. She came to see you after losing her husband in the same circumstances. My GP prescribed depression tablets but they are still sitting in my bathroom cabinet. I don't want to go that route. But I need to do something that is for sure. The path I'm on isn't a good one.' Jim suddenly buckled. 'Oh hell! I promised myself I wouldn't do this, make a show of myself... I need to man up!'

I waited while Jim paced the room, his hunched back turned. He stepped outside, wiped his eyes then came back to his seat, apologising profusely.

'Don't be sorry Jim, please. This is half the battle, sharing how you feel. We need tears to help us move through the strong feelings of our grief.'

'I guess you're right. I don't really know if you or anyone can help me. All I know is I have to try. Aileen would have given me a kick up the backside if she had seen me lately, moping around aimlessly. And she loved horses, she'd have liked me to do this.'

Finding safety

When we went outside, the herd of two we were working with grazed at the other side of the paddock. Beyond, the ripening crops glistened in the sunshine and further still the blades of an old windmill turned slowly in a light breeze. I could almost hear them creaking. Jim soaked in the scene and I noticed his breathing slow and deepen.

'They don't seem to want to know me,' observed Jim after he'd been standing near the horses here for a few minutes.

'What makes you say that?' I asked.

'I thought they might have come over to me. But they just want to eat.'

'And how is it for you, Jim, that they are not coming over?'

'It feels like I am on the outside, you know. Not really knowing how to approach them. Feeling awkward.'

'So, close your eyes and imagine a moment in your adult life when you felt most safe and most confident. Let the feeling live in your body, remember what it was like – the felt sense of it. Picture what you were doing and who you were with. Bring it alive. All the while taking the feeling of safety right down into your feet.'

Jim closed his eyes and I kept a watchful eye on the reactions of the horses nearby. They began to take an interest in him and soon Molly, who usually kept to herself, walked slowly over.

'Gently open your eyes Jim, taking care not to startle,' I guided.

'Oh! She's gorgeous!' The man began stroking her neck and fondling her shaggy mane. Her splendid moustache twitched in relaxation. 'Aileen would have so loved to be here.'

It was unusual for Molly to be the first horse to approach a new visitor, so I asked Jim what he had been thinking and feeling the moment before she had done so.

'It was on my wedding day. Aileen was on my arm, and I remember thinking how proud I was that she would be beside me forever. Well, I thought she would be ... That day I felt the safest I think I ever have, knowing we'd stick by each other. Life suddenly didn't seem as scary. And just now, remembering all that brought me this amazing feeling of calm. All the babble which usually drives me crazy, the what ifs and why didn't I's, I switched it all off. For the first time since she died I was quiet.'

'And can you go back there, Jim, when you notice that you are starting to feel lost again? Can you go back to your wedding day?' I suggested.

'I can, yes. Sometimes it's hard though to keep all the chatter out of my head.'

'Try imagining blowing all the thoughts which are plaguing you into a big balloon. Then tie up the end and let it float away.'

Jim looked at me sidelong, 'I will give anything a go once!'

Jim continued to come and chat with Molly over the coming months. Sometimes I would teach him ways of quietening his mind, but mostly he simply hung out with his hairy equine companion. She welcomed him always with the same docile sturdiness. He would lead her about the paddock, exploring the dandelions, seed-heads and grasses to see what she best liked to eat. Little by little he found his loss easier to discuss and began spending time again with the people close to him whom he had pushed away at the height of his mourning.

The day arrived for what would be Jim's final visit. Halfway through the session, he asked if he could take a break so he could return to the car.

'Yes of course, Jim. Is everything OK?'

'More than OK! I have to go to check on Prince. The dog I've just taken on. I heard he needed a home.' Jim's excitement shone. 'We're having some great walks together. Its getting me out and about to meet people. And it gives me a reason to get up in the morning. I couldn't always find it in me when I was feeling really bad ...'

I followed Jim to the car to meet the young, golden dog. I could picture the two of them on long walks, striding along riverbank and fell-side. Two lost souls who were finding a new rhythm together. As we both fussed over Prince, Jim cleared his throat:

'Coming here and working with you and Molly, it hasn't brought Aileen back. It never could do that. It has revived the self-confidence she gave me though. That is what has helped me the most.'

'Thank you Jim. It has been such a pleasure to see it returning, it really has,' I replied.

When we closed the session that day we agreed that now Jim would be able to continue building on Molly's intervention with Prince's support, but that he would call me if he needed to. I felt privileged to have been touched by the love he and Aileen shared which was still so vibrant. The window which Jim opened for me into the accepting, loving world of his marriage, challenged me to reflect on my own single status.

Could it be that I was missing something?

I heard some time later from Jim that he was doing well, although still with some way to go with his bereavement process. Prince's brother joined him too. A new family was forming.

15

Love

December 2015

Since arriving in Wiltshire I had continued to be single. The romantic disappointments of the previous decade left me with no appetite for building a new relationship. And besides, re-establishing myself and my business took just about all the creative energy available to me. I felt self-contained, independent and cheerful. Exposing myself again to the risk of heartbreak was not on my agenda at all.

Then my dog died. Holly was one of two Jack Russells I bought as pups. With her sister Milo, who had passed away the year before, she was at my side for just on 18 years, longer than any other living thing, bringing me light and comfort through the darkest of times. I had adopted another younger dog already, Maisie, but carrying Holly into my car for the final visit to the vet's was no less excruciating. In saying goodbye to her, I was also forced to confront in full the loss of her sister, whose essence had lived on with her litter mate.

Sometimes, when people ask me if I have children I reply 'Yes, but they all have four legs.' It usually raises a laugh and lightens the moment. My pets are the closest thing to kids I have experienced. Some might pity me, find it sad, emotionally unhealthy or anthropomorphic. Many understand the depth of attachment possible with a domestic pet. My life has been illuminated by the presence of my four-legged family members, canine and equine. The enduring inter-species understanding I have developed with each of them over long periods brings profound dimensions which I hold dear.

When I went home without Holly I felt utterly alone. Other bereavements were rekindled: my brother, parents, friends. Kind gestures and words were offered, but what I most needed was a hug and someone to sit beside me and share my sorrow.

I was no stranger to internet romance. I had previously been on dates (mostly just the one!) with men a foot shorter and a foot taller than me, with farmers and financiers, builders and beekeepers. There was the dinner with the son of a published culinary critic who complained about the perfectly acceptable food and wine and shouted at the chef 'You do know who I am don't you?' before he stormed out, and the meal with a landscape gardener which ended prematurely when I set fire to the tablecloth. He heroically threw the blazing fabric to the floor and stamped on it to quell the flames, melting the soles of his new shoes in the process. He didn't call me again. Then of course, there were the men for whom 'separated' meant still living with their wife but not having sex, and those for whom 'divorced' meant the ink was only just dry on the decree nisi and whose bile leeched from every pore.

Thus it was with an open mind and an attitude of curiosity that I sought once again to improve my love-life. My search was surprisingly short. A photograph of a Jack Russell who looked disarmingly like the dogs I had lost led me to John. Ten months after meeting for coffee one Saturday morning, he came to live with me.

16

Red Mars

Time to show

Every now and again, when work was quiet, and the weather too bad to be outdoors, when I was fed up with cleaning the house and I had already been out to my favourite coffee shop – in short, when I ran out of reasons NOT to open the document called 'My Story' – I would pick up the mouse and click. Sometimes I would write. Often I would simply read and marvel at the elasticity of time in which some events belonged to yesterday and others as if to another person completely.

Immersed in my writing I went to places inside myself I had never dared go, connecting differently to so many of my experiences. I noticed in particular how the life lived was often different to what I had shown the world at large. It was buffed up and presented so that the creases, cracks and downright pain of it were concealed. And here I was writing – in secret. Where was the authenticity in that? For someone whose livelihood revolved around helping others towards this goal, that seemed a bit rich.

And my story was nowhere near finished. Facing me that mountain to climb, that loss to deal with. The grief would boil up unexpectedly and wreak havoc like an unpredictable storm. Flashbacks to the intensive care room held me hostage at the most inconvenient of times. If I developed a temperature or showed minor cold symptoms my trauma whispered 'You could die too'.

To honour life itself, the one that I still was lucky enough to have, I understood that finish my book I must. To live by my espoused values of openness and authenticity, then *share it* I must. Continuing to hide parts of myself away was not an option. It was time for all of me to show.

The perspective of the planets

That evening I looked out of the upstairs window into the night sky which stretched above the gentle rise of Salisbury Plain. A red orb hung, bigger than a star, smaller than a moon, glowing faintly ochre. Red Mars. My brother Gordon was always obsessed with astronomy. 'You have to understand the moon, stars and planets, Pammie,' he used to say as I tried to slip back into the warm house from where he was glued to his telescope in the garden. 'They are bigger than us, bigger than life and death itself.'

Looking out on the awe which the red planet cast, beyond both my comprehension and my immediate emotional struggle, I finally grasped what my brother had been trying to tell me. The worries, even the grief, of my daily existence are not important, it is the universality of life, the vastness of what is possible, which counts. Here I was, my time on Earth slipping by, my potential limited by a need for parts of me to remain unseen. When out there, there was all this space available.

With this insight my perspective shifted. Gordon's life was so much more important than his death yet that was where my energy was drawn. His passing had become an ending. But now, with the Red Mars ahead of me, I pondered, perhaps it could be a beginning?

The next morning I stared at the blank screen where the next chapter needed to be. It was time.

I wrote 'Gordon' at the top of the page and started to type. It came like an avalanche throughout the day. I finished utterly exhausted.

Since Ellie died, I was a treasured friend to Dawn, the other Shetland. The new configuration of the herd of three, with Winston and Ruby forming a pair-bond, often left her without company. As soon as she saw me arriving she would trot over, her huge mane bouncing in rhythm with her shaggy legs, and position herself firmly at my side. She would shadow me as I worked, grateful at last for a companion.

So that evening when she ambled over to the picnic chair where I sat I wasn't surprised. Her sweet muzzle was knee height and she placed it gently in my lap with enough contact so that I could feel her breath through my jeans.

'I did it.' I said to her, cupping her flat cheeks in my palms. 'I went there and survived. I don't need to be afraid of it now. And maybe now I won't need to go back to that hospital room so often.'

As I stroked her elf-like ears her eyelids began to droop and, taking a few paces away she lay down to sleep. I moved my chair away and laid down beside her, matching my breath to hers. I found myself replacing the distressing images of my brother's body as his life ebbed away with ones of his laughter, his startlingly blue eyes and his quirky gestures. I imagined those images becoming bigger, as big as a house, so they blotted out the horrors which had been haunting me. His wicked humour, irreverent approach to authority and crazy inventiveness seemed to dance around me. The air began to vibrate with that formless sense of him which I had known as he died. My pony slept on.

17

Out of the Closet

May 2016

The political and economic environment was worsening. 'Austerity' had become the way of life rather than a short-term economic strategy. Private and corporate client bookings were petering out and the holiday period when organisations seldom commission work from companies like mine was yawning ahead of me.

In a chance conversation with a decorator I knew he mentioned that he was struggling to fulfil his order book and that it was impossible to find someone to help him.

'I'm good with a paintbrush, I'll help you out.' I quipped.

'Oh! Would you?' He surprised me by saying. 'That would be fantastic!'

I wasn't sure whether to be delighted or horrified. For a start my lines weren't that straight, but also, was this really the best way for me to be spending my time? After seeing the Red Mars I had spent days and days writing. I was on a roll, but there was still a long way to go.

'What is it going to be?' I asked myself. 'Are you going to take yourself seriously and at least show someone your book? Or are you going to spend the summer getting a sore neck from painting ceilings?'

In trepidation I spoke to a great friend who was the editor of a leading broadsheet weekend supplement. Apologetically I stuttered 'I've kind of written, a sort-of book … Would you have a quick look at it … only if you have time … I just want to know if its rubbish or if its worth carrying on? Be honest, don't spare my feelings.'

I didn't have to wait long for my friend to get back to me. 'Pam', she said. 'It's brilliant! It's just a first draft, I can see that, it needs a lot of work. But my advice is … go for it!'

The decorator wasn't surprised, but a little disappointed, when I called to say that I wouldn't be able to help him after all, that something else had come up.

I set to work. I was an author out of the closet.

18

A Team Embraces Vulnerability

They came from the heart of a sales driven organisation. A jumble of genders, ages, backgrounds and nationalities yet all senior leaders setting out to break the mould. They acknowledged that the management style which had served them for decades was no longer building the business, winning clients or motivating employees. Growth had been driven by pushing harder and squeezing more. Now they were committed to, quite simply, bring a human touch back.

Before embarking on the first interaction with the horses we had to subdivide the group of twenty into smaller groups of four in which they would be operating for the rest of the day. Five pairs of horses grazed each in their own paddock, and I asked the members of the group to gravitate towards the ones with which they felt most affiliation. With the rest of the team supporting me in the delivery of the programme I stood back and observed the process as the participants mingled. Several went directly to stand near their chosen horses without conferring with colleagues. A few others drifted from one paddock to the next looking lost, trying to decide which equine learning partners they wanted to work with. Yet most of the group quickly formed small huddles and bowed heads in hushed and frenzied discussion of which snatches could be heard.

'Let's get those two little ones over by the gate, they look easy!'

'The big black cob over there, he looks fast. Let's get him and his friend.'

'I don't like the look of that dapple grey one, he was the one standing in the corner before all by himself.'

'Let's try to get the pair of brown ones if we can, they seemed more interested in us and willing to cooperate.'

Winning habits die hard

Even though the group had voiced a desire for cultural change, it was clear that, at this stage, most had defaulted to a competitive mindset. With a few notable exceptions, the choice of which horses the women and men wanted to work with was based on a cognitive strategy aimed at 'winning'. Relationship had not come into it at all. Different theories were being aired about which equine qualities may or may not assist them in their quest to outperform their colleagues, which was essentially what most of them were aspiring to do.

When the two brown mares ended up with not one but two groups of four at the gate, arguing as to who got there first, I called time and asked the entire band of twenty to gather round me.

'Could somebody remind me why you are all here?' I asked in a neutral tone. Nothing. I waited.

'To build a leadership culture based on humanity.' A quiet voice eventually lifted from the back.

'Thanks, Fabienne,' I continued. 'Without discussing or commenting on this to your colleagues, close your eyes for a moment and consider what has been motivating you personally so far. Hold this in your mind, and notice the felt sensation of that intention in your body.'

I allowed a few moments to drift by, before inviting anyone who was willing to share their insights to do so.

Fabienne who had broken the silence earlier was first to speak. 'I wanted to work with the small ponies because I thought they would be more manageable and easier for us to control. I've tried to get a fix on how that made me feel physically. The interesting thing is that, I don't think I was feeling anything at all, I was mostly in my head, calculating how to convince the rest of the group.'

Wade spoke up next: 'I wanted us to work with the big black horse and his friend because they seemed to be the bosses in the herd. I thought that would help us to do well. I am aware of having felt quite singular in my desire to get them. That sensation is a familiar one, I hold my breath and feel tight and tense, like I want to punch my way through to what I want. Not literally, of course! And I realised how I lost awareness of everything and everyone else due to that focus.'

Relationship – a window to change

A hand went up from Toby, who was hovering at the back of the gathering. During the observation activity with which we had started the day, I had noticed how every horse investigated this man and offered him their nose. And when we broke out of the main group he had gone straight to the horses he felt drawn to, without concurring with anyone else: a young dapple grey gelding, Blue, and Ted, a huge cob with feathered feet the size of footballs.

'When we were observing the horses earlier,' he said, 'I loved it when each of them came up to me and just placed their nose on my hand. It was magic. I just wanted more of the same, so I chose the horse who had greeted me first, the grey one.'

I clarified, 'And when you arrived at the paddock with the grey horse, can you put any words around the felt sense of how that was?'

I saw his eyes glance across to the horse as he considered his response.

'I just felt happy. Nothing more complicated than that. It was an easy choice, I didn't have to think about it. I wanted to get to know them better.'

Toby captured the attention of the entire group with his words. The window to change had been eased open. This retiring, softly spoken man had made a heart-based choice motivated by a desire for relationship. Without any of the competition, the manipulation, or the tactics, he had already created, effortlessly, something special with his chosen herd. They were not a means to an end, or a tool in his armoury. They were living things with whom he wished to engage.

An attention to 'other'

While acknowledging Toby's contribution I took eye contact around the rest of the group, 'Now I'd like you to make your choice of learning partners again, this time by moving towards the horses you feel drawn to, not the ones you think will help you to win. Notice the felt sense of that experience physically and whether it is different or not to the one you had before.'

The group drifted slowly and thoughtfully back to the paddocks. Although the groups changed, as well as the atmosphere, there were still too many people gathered around the two gentle brown mares. I had to concede to myself that the pair of them were extremely beguiling, after all. A coin was tossed. Not exactly a relational process but consensual at least.

Throughout the day the pebble which Toby had dropped sent its ripples. Each small interaction between human and horse yielded further awareness. More quickly than I would have thought possible, ego began to lose its potency. Where an eagerness to do well (or to be seen to do well) had been clear in the morning, something different was emerging. Into its place an attention to 'the other', whether that was horse, human, colleague or facilitator, quietly crept. As the men and women became more conscious of their impact, kindness and compassion eased self-advancement out of the door. As this softening took place the herd blended progressively with their two-legged companions, no longer keeping their distance or looking askance with a suspicious eye. The response of the horses offered immediate positive affirmation to the group that their shift in attitude, and the power it held, was significant.

Trust unfolding

Day Two dawned. The moment when a group arrives on the second day of a programme tells all. Sleep allows a processing of conscious and unconscious learning. Gone now was the performance anxiety, the invisible badges indicating job title, length of service or seniority. They were no longer colleagues, rivals, bosses, even fathers, mothers, sons or daughters. They were themselves. It showed in the loss of edge, the gentle steadiness of eye contact, the leaning in when listening and the absence of banter. With these people the horses had already done a great job. I felt excited as to how the next eight hours might unfold.

Different groupings of four were formed and, using the learning from the first day, they were invited to meet with their new equine partners. They were to do this together, not one at a time as they had the previous morning, and without any structured guidance from the facilitators team. From where I stood I was able to see panoramically the playing out of this activity. People moved slowly, mindfully, mostly in silence. Most of all though, it was the horses who told me what was happening. Without exception they were at ease with their new visitors. There was no disruption to their energy, their level of comfort or their desire to engage. The participants were successfully attuned, to not only their four-legged companions but also to each other.

The willingness of the group to take risks no longer manifested in cocksure, sometimes fabricated, boldness and the ability to 'get the job done' before everybody else. It became about slowing down, stopping to reflect and communicate. They were noticing not only their own emotions but those of others. Hearts were opening, dilemmas and fears shared and feelings allowed voice. Standing together without judgement of each other had made vulnerability possible.

As the end of the programme approached I invited each small group to finish the day by presenting to the rest of their colleagues, via a ten-minute 'demonstration' with their horses, what they had learned and what they were proud of.

Toby's hand shot up. 'We'd like to go first if that's OK with everyone?' He was joined by the three other members of his human herd: boisterous Craig, who I recall had a penchant for high risk sports, Kwame, a measured, earnest character and Ita, a high-achieving business school graduate with designs on a chairmanship.

Murmuring to each other they slipped through the post and rail fence and sat in a circle in the middle of the field. Their learning partners carried on grazing, barely giving them a glance. It was as if everything around the four figures had stopped bar the flight of the wild birds and the passage of bees from one clover blossom to the next. Then one after the other, the two horses slowly yet deliberately drew towards the four and were soon nibbling on the grass around them. Several of my team had drifted to the spot to ensure the group's safety, as they all rested together in the most natural way possible. There was no touching, stroking or talking to the horses. Yet the depth of rapport was evident as the horses began to snooze beside them, feeling safe, welcome and calm. When Toby, Craig, Kwame and Ita broke away they were glowing with the light of interconnection.

No vulnerability, no change

I asked them later if they could define what it was the group had learned.

Craig spoke first. 'Trust has been a big issue for our organisation over the years. We decided to sit with the horses to show how easy it had been to develop trust with them, by being vulnerable. And how that helped us to open up to each other ...' His speech trailed off almost in disbelief at what they had achieved, he looked to his colleagues to continue. When Ita stepped in her words rang with what I could only describe as triumphant wonder.

'And wow! Did you see what happened? If we can achieve a tenth of what we built with the horses, with our teams, that would transform everything!'

They were right of course. Change is not possible without a willingness to take risks. And it was no different for me. If I was going to create change in *my* life, I had to do the same. If these men and women could embrace vulnerability, could I too?

Finishing my book, a memoir, and publishing it would expose my personal story, my hopes and fears, struggles and triumphs, beliefs and breakthroughs. It didn't get riskier than that. The part of me which really wanted to crawl back into my cosy shell sneered 'Who do you think you are? Who would be interested in what *you* have to say?' But the woman who wondered at the enormity of life's possibility before her, was growing in strength and said each morning 'Today I am going to be a bestselling author' before sitting down at her desk. Each time I did this I believed in myself a little bit more and took another small step towards creating a new reality.

19

Brittany

June 2016

It wasn't an ideal day to be walking on the beach. Cold rain blew horizontally across northern Brittany from east to west. We got the last available table at the restaurant, positioned by the window which was misted opaque with the breath of three dozen diners. As lovers do, we stretched the meal out with intense conversation, amusing each other with anecdotes, thirsty to know the other's history. I had already confessed to John my aspirations as an author. Whenever my confidence faltered he would just smile that smile of his, look at me with steady eyes and say 'It is amazing. Everyone will love it.' Our talk drifted to hopes for the future. I talked of writing, of continuing my horse-led work at my own place and living with my horses beside me. He of his desire for an organic smallholding, something he had come close to doing in Wales some years before.

Eventually the noisy clatter in the kitchens signalled that the staff were hungry and we were overstaying our welcome. The sky had cleared and the bright sun drew steam from the pavements and sand-flats. We strolled, hand in hand, along the shoreline and fell into silence. The sounds of the sea stroking the shingle and the wind in our ears was all the conversation we needed. John stopped in his tracks and turning, took my hands in his. His look unbalanced me. I got the feeling that he was going to say something big. An alarm rang loudly somewhere inside my head, and I pleaded silently 'No! Don't ask me that! Not yet! It's too soon!'

'We could live here, you know, in France.' Was what he said, instead. 'Both achieve our dreams. I could retire early. We could grow old together here. Why not?'

I was dumbstruck. Suddenly, this man I was growing to love was offering me the crown jewel of my dreams, wrapped in tenderness, adventure and presented on the finest cushion of burgundy velvet.

'What? Buy somewhere in France? And move? Together? Really?'

During the next few days, in cafes, on promenades, in bed, waking and sleeping we embellished in our mind's eye the ideal home and the lifestyle we could lead within it. An excitement started to build for both of us. It was sinking in that I would be fulfilling the commitment I had made to myself those years ago, without having to do it alone. I would have him at my side. The impossible had suddenly become infinitely possible in the most idyllic way. John was making a commitment to me and our shared vision. I flew as if on a magic carpet.

On the last morning of our holiday I woke feeling like I belonged to France already. I loved staying in this old manor house which dripped in tired elegance, spoke of minor noblemen, rich silks and damask and had glorious views of the trimmed topiary garden. My fluency in French was returning as I struck up conversation with anyone willing to engage (which is most people in rural France).

As I rubbed the sleep from my pillow-creased face I remembered. Today was the day. I didn't want to find out, I didn't want to spoil things, but I knew we wouldn't be able to avoid the news for long.

'You look!' I said to John. When he raised his eyes from his phone I knew.

'The vote is for Leave.' He was stunned, as was I.

Aside of my political view of the decision, which you can probably guess, I saw my personal goal and our recent plans, turning to dust. It was only in that moment that I understood just how much I had been thinking of this move over the past years. Emigrating in order to have my horses by my side, it had always been my 'get-out' clause. It had seemed like a fantasy, a distraction with which I entertained myself in dull moments at my desk or lonely bank holidays. But as John repeated, as if to convince himself that it was really happening, 'It's Leave. The vote is to Leave,' I realised that it was way more than that. Moving to France had become important. Removing this right, and my right to be European, against my will, felt totally devastating.

A sombre mood engulfed us for the rest of our day and the journey home. Where did this political decision leave our personal plans?

20

Unrest

July 2016

Even before the referendum took place the political uncertainty triggered by its approach impacted my business. Soon after the vote was announced two clients postponed large contracts and other events were cancelled completely. Therapy and coaching clients mostly stopped coming. The silver lining was that I had much more time to write, but this barely reassured me as I contemplated the long term economic climate.

Then came cause for optimism. I was invited to meet with a client based in London to discuss a long-term project for which we had designed and delivered a pilot programme some months earlier. It could be enough business to keep us busy for a couple of years. The feedback was overwhelmingly positive and I only imagined one outcome was possible from the rendezvous.

'You received the highest praise and scores we have ever seen for a pilot programme. Really, it was tremendous, you and your team are to be congratulated.' I couldn't help grinning as the compliments came. But as they say, pride comes before a fall. The programme manager lost eye contact awkwardly before continuing, 'Even so, I'm sorry to tell you that our purchasing department have found someone who will do it cheaper, so we won't be continuing this contract with you.'

I was speechless. The meeting took all of ten minutes, not long enough for the coffee I was offered to cool down. Out on the street in front of their prestigious offices I wondered why they had wasted my time, never mind the train fare, to tell me I was sacked. I was uncharacteristically incandescent.

When I arrived at the field the following morning I thought I had put my anger behind me. I lifted the huge tarpaulin sheet I used to keep the hay dry, loaded the wheelbarrow, ducked under the slip rail and set out to where the herd waited expectantly. Ruby, the most sensitive and least food-oriented of the three, flicked her ears back and forth quizzically, spun round and trotted pointedly to the furthest end of the five-acre field.

While I was scattering the hay I called to her. She looked in my direction, then turned her back on me. It was powerful feedback.

I am not my emotions

I checked into myself. What was happening for me right now to have caused this reaction? It wasn't difficult to work it out. I had been lost in the conversation of yesterday, what I should and shouldn't have said and done. I'd been wrapped up in negative emotions instead of being present in my body as I approached the horses. Inwardly I was ranting and brought with me, as a side-dish to the hay, a healthy portion of bad energy. The other two horses, well, their appetites always took priority. But Ruby, not her. She was demanding something different. I switched my phone off and placed a chair on the grass. I would sit and meditate until she came to me. Until then I knew I still had work to do.

Allowing myself to be with the emotions I had been feeling, I discerned so much more than the angry blaze which had ambushed me. Behind it was a sense of betrayal – we had delivered what the client wanted and beyond. I felt failure too

– why had I not seen this decision coming? And worry – was there going to be any more work out there for us? Not to mention outrage on behalf of my team who worked so hard.

Closing my eyes I let the sun touch all these feelings. I am not these emotions, I told myself, I can have them, let them go and still be here right now. This is a business decision taken by a man incentivised to cut costs. It does not change that what we did was good. It does not change who I am. I will learn from the experience and be available for the next opportunity which comes my way.

I don't know how many minutes later, a nicker from Dawn signalled the return of Ruby. I opened my eyes to see her shining form making its way towards me. She paused and I offered the back of my hand. She pressed her nose against my skin, as she does in her own special way, and joined the others as they ate. I was once more in my own world, calm and consistent.

An unexpected gift from a stranger

Courtesy of a faceless procurement professional, I was not short of time to spare. I took on the services of a writing coach. She told me that if I wanted my manuscript to be taken seriously it had to be at least 70,000 words long. I had a hell of a way to go. Yet the more I committed myself to the job in hand, the more passionate I became about it. The flow of consciousness which came when I connected with my experiences with a new eye was transforming my understanding of my work, of horses, of just about everything.

What I was doing by creating this piece of literature was beginning to feel important. Yet it wasn't sustainable within the structure of my current living arrangements if the economy continued shrinking. I talked it over with John. A financial case was building to support our venture. We decided to dip our toes in the water and a few months after our holiday in Brittany we booked a trip to France to go house-hunting.

21

Giving a Voice

September 2016

THE END.

I typed the words with a flurry and punched the air. I would learn later, as any experienced author will tell you, that completion of the first draft is the easy bit. But I didn't realise that then. Confronting the demons, traumas, disappointments and truths about myself I would have preferred to overlook was an emotional and physical endurance test. Crossing what I thought was the finishing line was a triumph.

Yet still very few people knew what I was doing. And now I found that saying 'I have written a book' in the past tense, felt even more fraudulent than saying 'I am writing' in the present tense.

Nonetheless and perhaps naïvely I began seeking an agent or publisher who would take me on. One after another rejection came. And often they didn't reply at all.

Months went by and my victory waned into despair. I'd walked blindfolded down a long tunnel with apparently no exit. What on earth had been the point?

The hoof

Then I held something in my hands which hauled out of me every last bit of determination at my disposal.

I'd signed up for a short course on hoof anatomy and how to maintain horses in good 'barefoot' condition (without metal shoes). Having been embroiled in my literary gloom, I was late in reading the joining instructions which I opened the night before the event. There was mention of studying 'cadavers'. Surely it didn't mean what I feared it might …?

The following afternoon, it lay in my lap. The lower leg of a medium sized pony collected from the abattoir that morning along with a few dozen others. Each wrapped in a bloody plastic bag. Some of the 'donor' hooves were in terrible condition, proof of neglect and untold suffering. And the stinking filth covering every specimen spoke of the degradation and horror they would have encountered in their last hours in the kill pens. But the foot I held, it looked healthy. Once this pony was loved and cared for. How did it come to end its life like that? The fur was dark brown, quite thick and slightly curly, the foot neat. It could have been from a native breed. Like Zeus.

Zeus, his image then came to me as strongly as if he was present. I sensed the intensity of his gaze, its mystery and healing. At the end of my tunnel I could see the light of purpose.

This was the point of my book. The potential of publishing. Through the pages I could speak for the voiceless horse. For every Zeus. For the pony whose foot I held in my hands. I could share with the world how worthy they are of our care and above all our protection. That they can make us more whole, more healthy, if we choose to acknowledge their nature. That their value goes far beyond performance and profit.

And, by publishing, readers who would never be fortunate enough to work with horses directly could share in the love and wisdom which I saw them bestowing on a daily basis. Even if my writing only improved one human and one horse's life then, surely, *that* was the point?

22

Guiseppe's Story

I now believed in the purpose of my manuscript, named *The Spell of the Horse*. The problem was that I didn't believe in myself as an author. Why would a literary professional give me the time of day when I couldn't even talk to my closest friends about my book without mumbling, squirming or making excuses?

A man called Guiseppe showed me what I needed to know. In his West of England accent, he told me why he came for coaching.

'I've worked my way up this company since I joined at 16. I am now 40. That is a long time. I'm a supervisor on the main logistics site where I have always been based. I love the company, but you know, I'm bored. I want more challenge. And … it feels disloyal to say it … but I feel my boss is holding me back. He never puts me forward for the managerial openings when I know I could do those jobs with my eyes closed.'

Guiseppe went on to describe how his manager often put him down in meetings, took credit himself for his supervisee's achievements and rarely gave him positive feedback. What was also clear was that the man sitting before me had had enough and was ripe for rebellion. Yet he also felt grateful to his boss who had recruited him all those years ago when apprenticeships were like gold dust. He was conflicted as to how he should proceed.

The football team

Outside in the paddock, the horses were uninterested in their visitor. Whatever he did to attract attention failed to make an ear twitch or eye blink.

'Can you think of a situation, Guiseppe, where you feel that people take notice of you? Where they give you your dues?' I asked, after he had returned to consult me despondently.

'Yes, when I am coaching the under 8s local football team. My son plays with them. They even do as they are told sometimes!' he offered without hesitation.

'OK so enter the field like you enter the pitch on your coaching days. Act as if the horses are three kids in the team. Command their attention.'

It took a moment for Guiseppe to conquer his shyness, but sure enough he swaggered back over to the horses, several inches taller, and called 'Fall in lads!' The three sets of ears trained on him left him chuckling out loud. The point was made.

'So, back at work Guiseppe, have an experiment,' I suggested. 'Take the same authority into every meeting as you do onto the football pitch. With your boss, his boss, anyone. Don't change anything else at all about what you do or how you do it. Just embrace your authority. It is rightfully yours to claim after so much experience with the company.'

I heard the advice I was offering him and realised wryly that I badly needed to take it myself. I may never have written anything before, but it was me who had lived the life I was describing. Surely I was the expert in that?

Finding authority

At his next session Guiseppe updated me with amusement.

'The funny thing is, I just pretend that the senior management are all kids I'm coaching. I even imagine them in their football kits. People are listening to me in a new way, it's incredible. I got a call last week from my boss's boss asking for my advice on a new system they are installing in our Swiss plant.'

'And your manager? How is he taking it?'

'I don't think he was pleased when the Director came straight to me, to be honest. But I was careful to keep him in the loop. I ended up feeling quite sorry for him. He's of an earlier generation and doesn't fully understand the potential of technology. I've realised he's just scared of losing his job. I'm trying to show him that I can help him stay in the game if he lets me.'

It was one of those occasions which I celebrate, when, after three sessions, Guiseppe called to say that he couldn't come anymore because he had been offered a short placement overseas, taking his wife and children with him. I congratulated him, and wondered, could I be as successful in embracing my authority as he had?

Stephanie – January 2017

As a first step I decided to participate in a one-day writing course in London. At the end of the day I said goodbye to one of the participants whose company I particularly enjoyed. I realised I didn't know anything about her. 'What do you do, by the way?' I asked. 'Oh, me? I'm an independent publisher,' she replied.

She was called Stephanie and several weeks later I signed a contract with her to publish *The Spell of the Horse*. There was no going back.

23

Dwight's Story

Dwight offered his three colleagues concise yet observant feedback following each of their one-to-one coaching sessions. When his turn came to work with the herd he seemed to shrink away when I invited him forwards. I softened my posture and let go of any sense of expectation, tilting my shoulder away from him slightly as I might when meeting a nervous horse. The space created released some pressure.

'I think I'm ready – as much as I will ever be,' he said.

We entered the paddock where the two bay rescued racehorses, Juniper and Paso, were relaxing some distance away. They nibbled on dandelion heads for entertainment rather than nutrition, their bellies already round and replete. The relaxation they emanated was in stark contrast to Dwight's palpable anxiety.

'Before we go any further, Dwight, can I check in with you on how you are doing?' I explored.

'I am pretty nervous, I can feel my legs shaking.'

'OK so first of all take some good deep breaths and feel your feet on the ground. And remember what I said earlier – there is no requirement at all for anyone to approach the horses, or do anything which feels unsafe, that is not the point of the work. The coaching can be equally successful outside of the paddock boundary.'

Dwight laughed almost scornfully 'Huh! The horses are the least of my worries. It isn't actually them I'm scared of. My sister had a pony when we were kids – I'm quite used to them although I don't actually ride.'

'Say some more about what troubles you, then,' I quizzed.

Ashamed of feelings

He inhaled deeply. 'I've always been uncomfortable to show my feelings. The thought of doing so terrifies me. This memory comes up of my Pa yelling at me for crying about something when I was young. He raised his hand, told me to be quiet or he'd really give me something to yell about. He never hit me, just used to make me feel very small. Don't think I have ever cried in public since. Stupid that it still matters so much.' The memory carried a biting energy which caught in his throat. He went on, 'People are always saying that they can't work me out, or that I'm cold.'

'And how is it to share this with me Dwight?' I asked gently.

'Weird!' And then he looked me in the eye for the first time. 'Strangely uplifting, too, which surprises me. I didn't think I had it in me.'

Horses don't need words

'The good news Dwight, is that the horses don't need you to say anything to know what your emotions are. They just sense them. And when we rejoin the group, there is no obligation to share anything which makes you uncomfortable. OK?'

He nodded and I continued, 'Approach the horses in your own time and your own way. There is no agenda other than for you to build rapport with them in this session. You can choose how to do that.'

Dwight paced slowly towards the horses. Juniper, the taller of the two, with kind eyes and ears which danced back and forth with curiosity, acknowledged his approach with a tilt of the head. Then in several trot paces he sprung daintily to

Dwight's side making contact delicately with his silken muzzle. Dwight smoothed both palms in a sweep down either side of the horse's slim neck.

'Shall we go for a walk, Juniper? What do you think?' And off they went, together, casually meandering around the paddock, the horse's nose tipped towards the man's chest.

Too soon the end of the session came. Dwight said goodbye to Juniper but when he turned to walk away the horse followed him back to the group.

When I invited Dwight to share what he wished to about his session he hesitated, looked at his colleagues and gulped air into his lungs.

'I was terrified of these two days. Not because of the horses but because I find it so difficult to express how I feel. At work I'm always receiving feedback that I am aloof or hard to fathom. But because I don't talk about my feelings it doesn't mean I don't have any ... When Pam said the horses would know how I feel without me having to say anything. It was like a weight being lifted ... Then Juniper came right over to me and just wanted to hang out, that blew me away. He even followed me back here! He must actually like being with me. I guess it has made me think if I could find a way to express myself maybe people would like me too.'

His colleagues recognised the gravity of this moment and felt no need to validate or comment on what had been said. Eyes betrayed admiration for Dwight and the emotional authenticity he displayed.

For the rest of the workshop, Juniper and Dwight were joined at the hip. It was endearing and sometimes comical to see them together. Even when Dwight was not involved in the sessions and stood at the fence observing the others, the horse's gaze would follow him. Under the reassurance of his equine teacher the man's defences slowly dissolved and a different person altogether began to emerge.

Set your beauty free

Dwight's experience with Juniper gave him affirmation that the emotions he had masked for so long were not only acceptable but also beautiful. Whilst Dwight knew that his difficulty in communicating originated from his early parenting, he had struggled to bypass the control which this experience held.

Shame starts as a small seed which is fuelled by our desire to stay safe and our need to belong. Sometimes a useful human emotion, it can motivate us to operate within standards which are considered to be acceptable within our society. The unpleasant physical feeling which goes with it indicates that we may have crossed some unacceptable boundary, perhaps one we weren't even aware of, and that as a result we risk being cast out. As an infant banishment by our care-givers is life-threatening. This is why we experience shame as one of the most visceral and terrifying of emotions, and why it is so debilitating when wielded as an instrument of control by those close to us. Shame, however, is not on a horse's spectrum of emotional experience. To them it is a false state of being. Thus, at their side, we can set free the beauty of what has been hidden behind it.

24

Two Into One

January 2017

It was really happening. Sometimes I had to pinch myself. My business was recovering with healthy bookings coming in, a publisher had offered me a contract and the man I loved wanted to live with me on a farm in France.

We hadn't found the right property but our visits were helping us clarify our requirements. On the first trip we wasted days and travelled hundreds of miles seeing unsuitable properties which were imaginatively described. We were learning that 'a little tired' could mean a house needed re-building, and the presence of an 'en-suite bathroom' didn't guarantee anything other than a toilet in the corner of the bedroom surrounded by a chest-high curtain. In planning the second and third visits we knew what questions to ask.

John sold his house and moved in with me, squeezing as many of his belongings into my small three-bedroom house as he could. The rest was stacked in my garage. He arrived after Christmas in a blaze of boxes, bookcases and ornaments I hated. Before I knew it my home was unrecognisable. Before he knew it, he didn't have one. He missed his own space and hated everything about mine. From day one it seemed that we had made a mistake and we were often irritable. We discussed renting somewhere bigger, in the UK, to ease the tension. But with the move to France on the horizon, what was the point? We decided that we could cope for the short term.

We were either planning our next house hunting trip or recovering from the last, that year. Life took on a transience and, other than work contracts, I felt unable to commit to long term scenarios. It became a little like riding on a roller coaster, with only rare opportunities to find my feet on the ground and stop the world spinning. I was working full-time on The Spell, discovering just how much I had to do before it was in a publishable state. Stephanie patiently supported me, through multiple cycles of re-structuring and editing. She shared her knowledge and expertise whilst allowing me still to own my work. The process was like combing a very large head of hair on a windy day trying to get the knots out.

Then one day, I realised that my manuscript had become like a large ball of plasticine which I knew inside out. I could shape it, mould it, stretch it, separate and recombine it with ease. The placement of each word, each sentence became an act of worship, bringing a centred tranquility rather than confusion and self-doubt. Finally, I was a writer. I embodied the authority which I had been honing over the past year. It came through sheer hard work and unbreakable commitment.

25

Doesn't Go

August 2017

Like so many of the others we had seen, the house could have been perfect. But there it was at the end of the sloping meadow. The road. Lorries hurtled by on their way to the motorway. Not even the immaculately renovated farmhouse, purpose-built stables or proximity to a delightful market town, could compensate. With heavy hearts we began the route back to Calais. These trips were costly in time and money. And when we got back, my house seemed smaller each time. We were both tiring of the search.

Sitting in my sun-drenched conservatory the following weekend we pored over our notes from all our property viewings of the past two years. There was only one place which both of us loved. We had dismissed it because the vendor was asking too much and hadn't been willing to negotiate. The house was still for sale. Maybe a year later, she might bend a little? I rang the agent who felt we stood a chance. We estimated the building works we'd need to do, calculated a sensible offer and reserved a cross channel tunnel weekend return.

'I think we'll change the gates, don't you?' I said as we pulled into the sweeping drive several weeks later. It was as if we already owned the house, which came with twenty-six acres of organic pasture and four of mixed, ancient woodland.

Swinging off the driveway into the neglected courtyard my bubble burst. The side of the stone barn had crumbled into a pile of rubble exactly where I would have stored my hay. The land looked as if it had not seen a tractor since our last visit a year earlier and ragwort, a weed which is poisonous to horses, was rife. Even before we went into the house and saw the damp patches on the walls, the water damage from loose roof tiles and the malodorous nicotine glaze on the beams, my stomach sunk into my sandals. Was it possible that an unloved property could deteriorate so much in twelve months? Significant investment would be needed to transform it into the nirvana we had been imagining. Neither of us had the appetite.

Back home, it was as if the bad energy of the house we'd intended to buy stuck to us like the tar which clung to the ceiling. It hung around, emerging persistently when I thought it had gone away. Things between us became strained and fractious. Other things were blamed, the lack of personal space, the long commute to work, the poor internet signal, the occasional noise from the neighbours. But something was changed. Something was not being said. Then finally it was out in the open. 'I don't want to go to France', he said. 'I'm sorry, I can't leave my family, or my job. And I need my own place, I'm moving out.'

He was right of course. We both needed to regroup. It seemed that two into one didn't go, after all.

26

Unravelling

We had viewed too many houses which were being sold by separating couples, with one partner loving France and the other hating it, for me to try and convince John to the contrary. It was different for him – he had children and grandchildren in the UK and a successful career in which he was still engaged. I possessed no such ties. I understood his decision but it was no less devastating. We'd built a clear plan for our future together. Now that was gone and my paradise with it. Sharing my home had become a source of unhappiness for us both so I felt some relief that he was moving out. Yet at the same time the sense of abandonment left me hurting and bewildered.

As our relationship faltered, I realised that we had become like a couple who spend a long time planning their wedding, obsessing about what colour serviettes they should have, instead of developing a shared understanding of the meaning of their commitment. Then, once their nuptials are behind them they have nothing to talk about anymore. We suddenly seemed to know more about the French property market than we did about each other. A gulf opened between us. If we weren't going to France, and we couldn't live easily under the same roof, where else was there for our relationship to go?

They say that fate gives with one hand and takes with the other. My precious book would be published in less than three weeks' time, but my romance seemed to be over and my vision to live in France destroyed.

27

The Launch

September 2017

To be seen above the crowd of chattering heads I created a podium out of boxes and draped it with cloth. The sides of the marquee magnified the buzz of animated conversation and echoed with the rise and fall of voices. Images four feet high of my beloved herd punctuated the room and brought the spirit of the horse in amongst us.

Climbing up to address the gathering I floated on a sea of love. People came from near and far, old friends I had not seen for a long time and new ones who I barely knew. None of them were aware how much I needed their support that evening, nor how grateful I shall forever be for having received it.

Publishing *The Spell of the Horse* was leaving me proud yet mostly terrified: of judgement, failure and ridicule. Through this memoir I was offering my soul up on a plate and I felt the most vulnerable I had in my entire life. At the same time, I was coping with the almost certain ending of my love affair and the curtailment of our emigration plans.

And here they were, my loved ones, bouying me with encouragement and reassurance. With their support I could bravely set The Spell of the Horse free. What I did not realise that night, as the heavens opened and the rain hammered on the canvas above our heads, was that the tricky thing with authenticity is that once embraced, as I had done through my writing, it prevents us from taking the easy road. Sometimes, it means we have to take the high one.

28

Dawn Meets Millie

November 2017

Constant companion

Since her identical 'twin' Ellie had passed away nine months earlier, Dawn had remained healthy. The loss of her life-long companion, however, left her solitary within the herd of three. The loyalty and affection formed between a pair of horses or ponies lasts a lifetime. Even those who are separated for many years will renew the pre-existing ties. She must have missed her field-mate terribly.

Age having stolen her teeth, Dawn needed many small meals of soaked hay nuts every day. I'd visit often and stay as long as I could. During these hours she became my constant companion waiting for the next serving and seeking companionship. In the milder months I would sit with her and she would snooze, with full belly and the sun soothing her old bones. If my garden had been bigger I would have taken her home.

Millie

John was preparing to move out and to give him some space I went away for the weekend. I should have known it would be dangerous to visit this riding buddy of mine who collected horses for a hobby. As we caught up on our news, I told her of Dawn's loneliness. Suddenly we were on the internet. A particular Connemara pony caught my eye, she was for sale not at all far from where my friend lived. The next day we went to meet her. She was called Millie.

There were more reasons not to buy this pearlescent beauty, than to buy her. She had a sore back and a sore mouth – I suspected poorly fitting tack and unsympathetic riding – and she was not used to living in a herd. Of course, these were also reasons why I couldn't leave her behind. I felt that mysterious heart-to-heart tug take place between us. The one which I have experienced when all my horses and ponies have chosen me for themselves. Two weeks later she was delivered. She had been separated from the half-sister she'd spent her whole life with and the emotional impact was significant. But Millie and Dawn found instant solace in each other and became inseparable. Millie would shepherd her small friend around, shielding her from Ruby and Winston as if she were a foal.

Something wrong

On a cold, wet morning three weeks later, instead of tucking into the feed I had placed in front of her, Dawn followed me as I walked away. Puzzled, I offered her the bowl again. She buried her muzzle in the mushy substance, but as soon as I made to leave her soft nose glued itself to the back of my knee. There was no doubt she wanted to come with me. I slipped the rails and led her up to the field shelter, out of the wind and rain. I fetched more feed, hay, water and a rug to warm her up. She started to calm down and set about eating. I spread a rug on the dry earth and sat down to monitor her for a little longer. I watched like a hawk for signs of further improvement. My heart soon sank. She stood. She lay down. Stood again. Walked in a circle. Her agitation grew. She couldn't get comfortable, couldn't keep still. I knew something was horribly wrong.

The vet came. She was kind. It appeared that there was nothing to be done. Certainly nothing which I wanted to put an old pony through. A sedative was given which eased the pain and I had to smile as Dawn began tucking into her breakfast bowl with gusto. She ate until her eyes drooped sleepily and passed away peacefully under the distant gaze of Millie, who called from the other end of the field.

Dawn had lived happily, there was no tragedy in her passing. Simply, I missed her and the joy she brought me. Her gentle and assured presence, the way she waddled after me, the huge whinny heralding my every arrival, the nickering which escorted me on my chores and the precious unicorn's head peeping through the fence to greet me.

Millie missed her too. She was doubly bereaved. Her emotional turbulence manifested in acute reactivity to the other two horses who were keen to maintain clear boundaries within the hierarchy. She'd burst through the electric fencing, run me down and once even jumped out of the field over the five bar gate when she felt too much pressure from them. It became difficult to manage her and soon it was going to get a lot worse.

29

The Winter That Was

Powered by a ferocious wind the snow stung my face as I hauled water from my vehicle. The horses' automatic trough had been frozen for days and was filled with a cubic metre of ice. I came three times a day with two ten litre containers which I filled at the tap in my neighbour's shed. What I was leaving would be frozen within the hour and I hoped the horses would drink before it did.

Arctic weather patterns brought twelve weeks of snow, ice, rain and freezing temperatures. The weather forecasters had christened it 'The Beast from the East'. I cancelled client sessions and there was no sign when I would be able to rearrange them. My hay was running low and I couldn't imagine how a truck was going to get up the long farm track with further supplies. Every muscle in my body ached from clearing snow, carrying water, shifting wet hay. The facilities at the field I rented were woefully inadequate. As I grumbled to myself my feet shot sideways in the mud landing me square on all fours. I'd have laughed if I hadn't been so miserable. Kneeling in the mud, I yelled into the storm 'I can't do this anymore!'

Coping with Millie was particularly difficult with the conditions underfoot. She didn't have the regard for me, the desire to keep me safe that Winston and Ruby possessed. They would step carefully around me, walking slowly if I had to lead them and even allowing me to lean into them for balance. They seemed to recognise my two-legged fragility. Millie however would pull away or push into me, spinning and leaping into a gallop if the others came near. More than once her flying hooves spattered me with dirt as she left. In different circumstances there was much I could have done to help her relate to me better. But now I simply had to leave her to her own devices and handle her as little as possible.

For the first time ever, I wasn't enjoying my horses. My passion, my pleasure and my emotional salve had become an ordeal. While my neighbours were staying safe and dry, I was sliding across the ice, on foot or in my car, trying to reach the herd to feed and water them. Sometimes kind friends helped me penetrate the drifting snow. But most trips I did alone.

Something has to change

Later on, as I toasted myself in front of the wood burner, I did what I always do when in need of counsel. I sat down with pen and journal and began to write. Had I relinquished my dream too readily when John pulled out? Perhaps, in a way, it suited me to believe that it was no longer possible? The prospect of leaving this place where I felt safe was frightening, there was no doubt about that. But was that all which was stopping me?

The idea of relocating abroad had been this golden glow on the horizon for a long time. It was my 'get out of jail free card' which I drew from my pack whenever down or frustrated. 'Never mind Pam, it will be alright when you live with the horses. It will all be better when you move to France' I'd say, patting myself on the head. As long as it was all just a fantasy, there was always hope and optimism. Yet if I turned my hopes into reality and it *didn't* make me happy after all, then where would I be?

Was it possible that my fear of failure was bringing more influence to bear on my decision not to go than I liked to admit?

What is *really* holding you back?

Something else surfaced as I scribbled. To resurrect the emigration plan on my own, well that would also mean stepping into an even bigger version of myself than I already had. I would have to fully embrace my power as a single woman, setting out to lead the life she desired. Was this, perhaps, the step which felt way too much to take?

I looked outside at the horizontal white-out which was again silencing everything but the wind. I had just an hour before the next visit would be needed to tend to the horses. Enough was enough. I sat at my computer, logged on, and opened a search for a property in France.

The harsh winter would continue for two more months. A severe chest infection left me shivering in bed for days and weakened for several weeks. The struggle that was caring for my horses worsened with this ill-health. Finding a new home for us was no longer a pipe-dream. It became a matter of survival for us as a unit. I knew another winter like this could see the end of me keeping horses completely. And what would my life be without them?

Horses open up a world for me, one of growth, joy, contentment, learning. They led me to my current way of working and to a nascent career as a writer. Our legacies were so intricately bound that living without them was inconceivable.

It was decided, I would relocate on my own. And I was going to be sure to achieve it before next winter came.

30

Steve's Story

We watched the three horses make their way to the water trough, undulating tails in fluid S shapes. Their gait rhythmical, contented, harmonious. The older horses allowed Millie to drink simultaneously to them, and they stood together, heads low in relaxation, water dripping off their muzzles in shining droplets.

I knew that Millie had struggled to adjust to her new life, particularly after the passing of Dawn. As the newcomer and least dominant member of the herd she was excluded by the other two. In the harshness of the winter when resources were scarce they would drive her away from food and water. She was as a result defensive, sometimes wild and difficult to handle. The chemistry we had shared when we first met disintegrated as conditions had worsened. In a field where I could barely stay upright for the mud or ice there was little I could do to build bridges with her. The scene now was so different.

The herd finds harmony

'Don't they look wonderful,' observed Steve. 'Like a wave flowing down the track. They all get on so well together. So harmonious.'

I pictured the scene a month earlier, the conflict amongst them, and how wary I was of Millie, and smiled to myself. What a transformation was taking place.

'What does harmony mean to you right now Steve?' I opened.

'Huh! I'd like a bit more of it!' He exclaimed.

Steve told me how he had taken on a new role as a director on the board of a small charity a year earlier. There were difficulties between him and some members of his team. He'd been offered coaching to help resolve them.

'I am beginning to regret taking the job at all,' he concluded. 'I'm not getting on with two of my four direct reports. They manage two thirds of the organisation, both staff and volunteers, between them so it is important we can work well together. But the harder I try to understand them the worse it gets.'

The herd were moving towards their hay which was spread out in piles. Millie was first to arrive. We watched as Ruby chased her off the first mound she stopped at and Winston chased her off the second. The two older horses moved her round, nipping at her rump if she disobeyed. Eventually, she was allowed to rest and eat and the three of them returned to amicable companionship.

'Oh! That's not so nice, is it?' exclaimed Steve. 'Poor Millie.'

'What did you see change Steve, in that little episode?' I asked.

'After they chased her off the hay a few times, they let her settle. I noticed that at first when they approached her and she didn't move, they bit her. Although it looked more like a warning than seriously hostile. But when she moved away immediately, they then let her get her head down to eat.'

'Well observed. Their behaviour is about respect within the hierarchy. The two older ones demand it from the youngster. They insist that she obeys their requests to move out of their way. As the junior member she has to yield to them. If she doesn't there are consequences, consistently applied. It looks mean, but it is really just about setting boundaries. Once those

105

are established within the herd, they can all relax and live together without friction.'

'Now it is sounding much more like the human world I am operating in!' Steve said with humour.

Establishing boundaries

Handing him a long piece of rope I asked that he create his own metaphorical boundary by placing it around him in a circle. A space large enough for him to feel like he is looking after his own safety, but not so big that the two of us couldn't communicate. He laid the rope down on the ground, stood in the middle and adjusted it until he was happy with the positioning.

'Do you feel safe and contained in there, in your personal bubble?' I asked and, while he was still nodding consent, I stepped forward without warning across the line. He looked startled and stepped backwards over the rope boundary behind him.

'You got me!' Steve was giggling while he lifted his hands in defeat.

'What feels familiar about this situation?' I looked out at him from within his circle that I had claimed for myself. The exercise had brought levity, now it was time to get serious.

'I tend to be the one who accommodates others. Particularly if they take me unawares. Although even if I am able to plan for a negotiation or tricky meeting I'm not much better at holding my position. I rehearse scenarios and difficult conversations endlessly, keep myself awake at night doing it, but I still cave in.'

'Is it possible that this pattern has been playing out in your relationships with your new team members Steve?'

'Yes, I guess it is. They take little notice of me and carry on doing their own thing. Then in little ways they undermine me by being late or leaving meetings early. I don't feel I can throw my weight around because they know the business so much better than I do. I need them on my side. I'll feel happier about challenging them when I fit in better.'

'Well, there is a difference between throwing your weight around and asking for their cooperation. And fitting in – there is a responsibility on both sides to enable that to happen.'

As I finished speaking, I noticed that Winston was moving towards us at a gentle, but seemingly unstoppable, pace. As he neared Steve he didn't slow down and moved the man aside decisively then turned to investigate him.

Steve was amused. 'There is a bit of a theme developing it seems!'

I handed the man a short lead rope and demonstrated how he could protect his personal space by swinging it gently around his torso from side to side should Winston try to invade it again.

'But I don't want to hit him!' he protested.

'You are not hitting him with the rope Steve, you are simply swinging it within the boundary of your personal space. If he chooses to walk into it then that is his look-out.'

Boundaries and trust

Before too long, the head of the herd once again decided to put the visitor to the test. Steve started swinging the rope and before Winston reached it he stopped dead and pricked both ears forward with interest.

'OK, so now walk towards Winnie, still swinging the string. You are only doing to him, what he did to you just a minute ago, and what he has been doing to Millie all afternoon,' I guided.

Steve walked forwards slowly, the rope swirling. Winston moved graciously away before the soft cotton made contact with his shoulder.

107

'I can't believe that just happened!' grinned Steve. Winston was now facing him and slowly turned his body so that it was sideways on. 'Now what on earth is going on?'

'He is asking you to scratch him, here at the base of his mane, like this. Its what horses do to strengthen their relationships. We call it mutual grooming. You have just shot up in the rankings from junior member to someone he wants to bond with.'

'Really? Amazing!'

While an ecstatic Steve was scratching Winston, I noticed Millie drift over and watch the proceedings cautiously. When Winston moved away, she sidled over to Steve, with the same request.

'This is too much,' he giggled, and rubbed her too until she wandered back to the hay.

Continuing with the exploration I asked Steve to mark his personal bubble on the ground again. He gathered the rope out of the dust and spread it out. I took two forceful steps towards him, but before I could cross his line he stepped forwards, lifting himself taller and stopping me in my tracks.

'How can I help you Pam?' he smiled assertively. 'Please, step into my office!' With an ironic flourish he stepped back making space for me on his side of the rope.

Creating a safe space for dialogue

Steve had learned that fitting in at the new organisation wasn't about bending to everyone else's demands and allowing them to transgress boundaries. There were power games taking place in the same way that they did within the herd. As leader, it was up to him to set the boundaries and thus make space for dialogue. The quality of both would dictate the leadership culture he could generate. When Steve reinforced his authority with Winston, the horse was then able to have a conversation about what he needed, and ask for something in return. Millie had followed the example. It would be no different at work. By establishing his leadership with clear boundaries, Steve wouldn't be closing people down, he was opening up a safe space for conversation. He was making it possible for his team members to ask for what they needed from him, and he could do the same.

A lesson in belonging

After Steve left I went back to sit with the herd for a while. How easy they are now together, I pondered. Between the three of them things are clear. While learning to fit in with the hierarchy, Millie is discovering how to ask for what she wants both from the other horses and from the humans she interacts with. By doing so she is finding a way to belong.

I was reminded of how long it takes to find one's place. That the process of fitting in happens organically. If I proceeded with my plan I would soon be uprooting myself and starting again, in a different country with little or no existing support network. I'd spent five years building a good life in Wiltshire. Would I regret walking away from it all? I felt acutely conflicted as to what I should do. It wasn't even head versus heart. It was as if my heart was split in two, one side wanted to stay, the other wanted to live my dream.

31

The House with the Red Shutters

July 2018

The red shutters and doors which had winked at me from the computer screen looked just as inviting as I pulled into the driveway. I was shown around the house which came with five acres and was situated in Mayenne, the region where my friends had settled. The farmhouse kitchen with its table seating eight, double aspect windows and door opening onto a wisteria-draped courtyard, chimed with a picture I had held since my youth. Then I'd imagined growing up to raise a chaotic family on a farm somewhere, with dogs running around and ponies out in the paddock. I could already hear the chatter of visitors gathering to share this welcoming space.

The rest of the interior left me ambivalent – it was badly renovated and needed modernising. But when I stepped outside into the garden, that was when I knew. The land fell away from the house and ended at a stream. The soft sound of running water from the spring beside the well-tended vegetable bed invited a long out-breath. Trees lined the perimeter of the land with birds darting from one copse to another. Chaffinches nested noisily in the grapevines around the patio. The impact on my soul was immediate.

Then I found the jewel in the crown. A large, old fashioned but immaculate hay barn adjacent to a small cow shed. The original hand-made wooden hay racks, eating troughs and even the names of the heifers, last resident in 1970, were still in place. An interconnecting door between the buildings meant that in winter, whatever the weather, both I and the horses could stay warm and dry, and in summer cool and out of the heat.

The rest of the property became immaterial. If it worked for the herd, I could make it work for me. This was it.

A few days later negotiations were complete, the vendors being as keen to move before winter as I was. That concluded, I began to tackle the backlog of emails which had built up during my absence. There was one onto which I whisked my computer mouse above all the others.

Good fortune

'I am delighted to tell you that we wish to go ahead.' I read.

A simple one-liner. Confirming that my company was selected to deliver a significant leadership development programme for a global organisation. It would span two or three years. I submitted a proposal a long time previously and was not at all sure if it would go ahead. My leadership development approach, centred on learning through mindful interaction with horses, although highly effective was often seen as 'off the wall' when compared to traditional approaches. But here it was, a contract bigger than I had hoped for.

Two days later, another email arrived. More work for the following winter was confirmed with a different client, and a third project was secured a couple of weeks after that. I laughed out loud. Famine for so long, and now that I had agreed a date to move to France, work for my company in the UK started flooding in. It was just as well I would not be too far from the ferry ports.

Attracting abundance

I didn't know what to make of this good fortune. I sensed that the transformation process I was embarking on was unlike any other I had experienced. My actions pulsed with the positive energy of vision and passion, whereas previously life-changing decisions had been about turning things around or rescuing myself from a toxic situation. For the first time I was seeking change in a strongly intentional way, rather than because circumstances were forcing it upon me.

I had seen around 30 properties. Each visit that Spring and Summer had made me more determined to move. John himself often accompanied me on the trips, offering assistance with the driving and buildings advice. We had recreated a friendship on the ashes of our heady love. His blessing felt important. Through these months, my self-belief had grown, fuelling a sense of empowerment and excitement. Could the change in my business's fortunes be an indication that this positive energy was attracting the abundance flowing my way? By taking a risk with my own life, were others now willing to take a risk on me?

32

Meg's Story

Within minutes of entering the paddock Meg's high-end hiking jacket was covered in a mixture of chewed grass and horse spittle. I made a mental note to include something about wearing washable garments in my joining instructions. AD, a mare whose aura filled the valley, wanted to play and she was particularly interested in the toggles on Meg's coat.

'It's a mixture of curiosity and jealousy which has brought me back,' she said. 'When I came to the open day with one of my colleagues last year the horses were all over her, every one of them! I was so envious. They all gave *me* a wide berth. I'd like to explore why that was … The learning could be useful to me. I will be retiring soon and am asking myself a lot of questions about what to do next.'

AD's reaction to Meg could not have been more different to what she expected. Very quickly the large, three-year-old mare became bored with the fastenings and focused her teeth on the beautifully quilted pockets instead. At that point I intervened.

'I'd like to step in for a moment Meg and help you and AD interact more safely, if that is OK?'

'Well, no it isn't OK, really, I am fine. I am just so relieved that she likes me.' I was a little surprised at Meg's response but signalled acquiescence.

AD seemed to have understood the exchange between us and began tugging on the fabric so firmly that she pulled the woman off balance.

'That showed me didn't it!' Meg said good-naturedly. 'I give in and bow to your knowledge Pam.'

I showed Meg how to maintain a safe distance between the rather large wandering teeth and the peached cotton garment. Very quickly the mare understood what was needed from her and settled into a more respectful interaction with her new partner.

Playing again

Soon Meg was moving her four-legged friend around like a confident professional. I pointed to a number of poles and blocks which were lying on the ground, the kind which can be used to construct small obstacles for horses, dogs or humans to jump over.

'See if you can find out how AD would like to play with these.' I suggested. 'You two seem to be on the same wavelength.'

Meg began tapping on the sticks and blocks. 'What would you like to do with these, AD?'

The mare locked her eyes onto Meg but for the first time stood still.

'What?' Meg faced her, hands on hips in mock reprimand. 'Come on, don't expect me to come up with all the ideas! Oh! I'm going home if that is the best you can do!'

Meg began to walk theatrically away until AD sprang forwards and overtook her in less than four canter strides. Meg's delight came from that spontaneous, uninhibited place many adults have forgotten as the horse landed in front of her. Meg turned on her heels, ran towards the poles and jumped over the ones which were flat. AD followed suit.

'Oh my! That is the most fun I have had in a long time!' Meg's words whooshed out of her.

114

At that point AD looked across at her field mates and began yawning. She was ready for a break and her disengagement confirmed that the work for the day was done.

Dutiful daughter

In the cosy classroom I began wrapping up the session. 'Before we explore what happened Meg, I'd like to sit for a moment, close your eyes, stay with the energy of your interaction, let it settle into your bones. Feel it flowing through your limbs, outwards from your belly and ending right back down in your feet. When you are ready, open your eyes and share with me what you would like to about your time today.'

In a little while Meg began: 'I was a serious child. Always on my best behaviour around my parents. They were quite strict. I learned recently it has a name – the Dutiful Daughter phenomenon. I think I learned it from my mum, she had it drilled into her too as a child. It never really wore off. Except when I was with Franny, my partner for 20 years. She knew how to make me lighten up. We used to have so much fun … I have barely laughed since she died three years ago. Until today.'

The heaviness of loss filled the room and I allowed a silent space into which Meg's memories and the spirit of her soulmate could come.

'Tell me what you loved about Franny.'

'Ah, her naughtiness. Definitely. When I was playing with AD I felt like I was playing with Franny. Maybe I was, who knows? I wouldn't put it past her to find a way of coming back to me. She had the same kind of charisma as AD too – she'd walk into a room and everyone would look round and smile whether they knew her or not.'

Sorrow resonated around us. Outside AD grazed, a comforting sight.

115

Friends reunited

'I think she recognises me!' cried Meg when AD trotted over at the beginning of their second session. The weather was more clement so thankfully there were no toggles to chew on.

The woman immediately asked AD to take a few steps back and the mare obliged. They walked together and played with the jumps as before, co-conspirators, startlingly familiar. Their rapport would be the envy of many a horse owner I reflected. Quietly from a distance, I observed this union of beings. Then AD began moving more slowly before coming to an abrupt stop. She yawned, relaxed one of her hind legs and adopted a snoozing position. Meg placed a hand on her neck and, without pausing, turned and walked briskly back to me.

'How are you doing, Meg?' I said softly.

'She seems to have had enough. I thought I'd give her some space. Shall we go back in for coffee?' Her tone was brisk, businesslike, the energy a little spiky.

'It does seem a good place to break, but I'd like us to stay a few moments with AD if that is good for you? When a horse is sleeping they like to have one of their herd mates somewhere near them. Her two friends are way over there. To stay and watch over her while she rests would be something special you can do for her.'

Meg agreed and took up a position around six feet from the mare whose eyelids were closed and bottom lip hung loose. Minutes went by then AD swayed a little and for a moment I thought she might lay down in front of us. Instead, she stretched her back like a cat and reached to nuzzle Meg's sleeve before departing. The work, again, was done.

Regret

Back inside the classroom Meg nursed a hot drink in her hands. Before words could come, her body folded into its pain.

'There is no need to say anything, Meg, unless you want to.' I reassured. 'A meaningful conversation has taken place between you and AD. That in itself is enough. If it helps to talk about it that is fine, but it is also OK to leave it unsaid. Sometimes human words are inadequate.'

'No. It is important that I speak this, it has been festering for so long. When Franny was ill ... having the chemo, I should have stayed with her. But I carried on working full time. I hate myself for it. I suppose I couldn't bear to see her so ill. It wasn't until the very end, when she was too poorly to enjoy having me there, that I took compassionate leave. I will never forgive myself, never. I walked away from Franny when she needed me, just like I left AD a few moments ago.'

Self-recrimination and regret leached with every word. 'The truth is I didn't know how to handle her illness. Every time I looked at her it hurt, knowing that she would die. Every moment we had, everything we did, was a goodbye. I couldn't bear it, so I avoided it. I let her down so very badly. And before I realised, it was too late. She was gone.'

The anguish was like grey, cold seawater, sweeping life before it.

'Do what you can to breathe Meg. Imagine Franny here with you now, with her arms around you.'

The storm gradually passed leaving a stillness.

'If it felt comfortable for you Meg one day, I would like to suggest that you write to Franny. You told me about the tree you planted together to mark your anniversary before she became ill. Perhaps sit beneath it on a pleasant day, take out your pen and paper, write about your feelings. Know that she will hear and respond.'

'I will, thank you.' Then, Meg smiled. 'I feel as if Franny was speaking to me through AD, reminding me not to be such a miserable old bag! She never did mince her words you know.'

117

Forgiveness

Several weeks before I left for France, Meg and I worked with the herd for the last time. A freshness came into the classroom with her, a brighter light shone in her grey eyes.

'I wrote a letter to Franny,' she began. 'It helped me to realise how angry I have been at myself for letting her down. And that I was mad with *her* too. For dying on me. How stupid! Like she had a choice. I'm finding a way to forgive both of us now. I just hope she knows it, wherever she is. If only we could have come here together. With the help of the horses we might have talked about what was happening. She might have been able to ask me to give up work. I would have done, at the drop of a hat.'

'Was that unusual for her Meg? Did she have difficulty asking for her needs to be met at other times?' I clarified.

Meg guffawed. 'She certainly did not! She was the opposite to me. Her family were tactile, caring, demonstrative, but also able to have a good rant. They never held grudges and always hugged after a row to put things behind them. She was a master communicator. Took me to task many a time.'

'Is it possible, I wonder, that she didn't *want* you to stop working? And that is why she didn't ask?' I ventured.

'Hmm.' Meg mused. 'I guess it could have been easier for her to carry on as normal. She needed lots of rest too, during the treatment, so may have needed the time alone. She left her affairs very tidy, which must have taken some doing. She commented once how time consuming the business of dying was. And she often scolded visitors if they got maudlin. She'd say her illness hadn't changed who she was or how she wanted to be treated.'

Space for a new kind of life

Although Meg was becoming more comfortable talking about her loss, when she did a part of her went somewhere else. I suggested that we go outside where I hoped that amongst the horses, enfolded by nature, she would be able to come back to herself.

Soon AD came to greet her, accepting long strokes on the neck. But she took herself away quickly, leaving the woman alone in the lush expanse of grass. Molly, however, the much older matriarch of the herd who had previously taken no interest, ventured a little closer. Thirty paces away she stopped, turned her shaggy black and white flank to the sun and began to toast herself gratefully. Meg sat down on the turf without closing the gap between them.

Many minutes passed. Nothing yet everything happened. Eventually Molly stretched and ambled to her human companion who caressed her muscled shoulder gently.

'That was different wasn't it?' Observed Meg as Molly withdrew. 'Not what I expected based on the other sessions.'

'Tell me some more about what happened Meg ...' I coaxed.

'I sat there after AD had wandered off. I wasn't disappointed funnily enough. I was thinking of Franny. The thought of her made me smile inside. And although I felt that ache which goes with losing a person you love, it wasn't with the desperation I usually know. And having all that space around me, I felt that AD was showing me I would be alright on my own. Then Molly came up, and I realised that, even without my wonderful partner, there is still so much happiness to be seized. It was like Molly was reminding me just to be me. I don't need to be the career woman anymore. I can retire from my business without losing any of my identity. I will miss Franny to my core, forever. But now I feel it will be possible for me to live a new kind of life when I retire, without her. Whatever that might mean.'

Meg put aside the guilt she'd carried for so long. She forgave herself and her soulmate. She had found a way of accessing her deepest feelings with the help of the horses, and of allowing them to move through her body. Healing had begun.

Two years later I had the opportunity to talk with Meg. She was retraining as a psychotherapist, and was shortly to fulfil her lifelong desire to have a dog. She radiated presence and there was an unmistakable glint in her eye.

'Being with AD and Molly reminded me of this golden time when my father was alive and he used to take me for riding lessons every week,' she recalled. 'He would sit and wait for me all afternoon. My mind had almost blotted out the happiness of that era, before I became an anxious teenager and adult workaholic. It has been so good to be reminded that once I wasn't like that.'

Living life in colour

'How has that helped you Meg?' I prompted.

'Something massive shifted in the months after my work with AD and Molly. It was almost as if *all* my feelings found a way to be free, to be accessible. Not just my sadness. And in experiencing my emotions more vibrantly I have been able to make better decisions. Giving up work was one. Training as a psychotherapist another. I have started running too! Unbelievable as I had never even worn a pair of trainers before. I am meditating and eat a more healthy diet. It's hard to describe the enormity of what those dear, dear horses have done for me ... it is like I am seeing myself in colour. Before I met Franny I lived in black and white. I wonder if that is one reason why I took her passing so badly, because when she died, the colourful version of me went with her.'

120

Hearing about the cascade of change which AD and Molly had initiated for Meg brought a sense of the enormous privilege of being party to such things.

'And what will you call the puppy?' I asked.

'Maddy,' replied Meg.

33

Continuity of Love

September 2018

Meg had described how every moment in the last months with her partner felt like a goodbye. I became aware that, whilst my circumstances were incomparable, I was seeing my own life in Wiltshire through a similar lens. I savoured every good experience, then dreaded leaving it behind. I was unconsciously bringing a veil down on the life I was leading. I was robbing myself of the joy which was still there for the taking in the here and now. I recalled the image of Meg sitting in the field, with a great green space around her, exuding serene hopefulness and I took inspiration from her.

Holding balance through change

The machine that is house moving had a momentum of its own. A sale was secured on my house, removals and horse transport booked, multiple trips made to charity shops with useful clutter and clothing. I lived in a permanent state of anxiety, every nerve buzzing under my skin. I repeated affirmations to help me hold my course: 'Nothing is forever', 'Trust the process', 'Be guided by the horses'. My nights were restless and my emotions fragile. Except when I was with the herd. Then it all made sense.

One evening in early October, two weeks before my departure, I pushed the barrow piled high with hay across the

122

grass. After spreading it in piles I paused. It was one of those magical evenings when you can see the sun setting and the moon rising at the same time. The world was held in balance between these two great orbs, on the cusp of the soft light of the day and the sharper luminosity of night. As I confronted the huge change I was facing, I wondered, could I hold myself in equilibrium in this way between my two worlds – the known and the unknown. Two stages of my life were waxing and waning like the sun and moon, one passing into the next, with no end and no beginning.

The presence of those we cherish

I brought my awareness to Winston, Ruby and Millie. Not so long ago, there had been Ellie and Dawn here too. Recalling the effervescent energy of the two small ponies brought a smile. How present they still felt when I closed my eyes and conjured every detail of their physical selves. I tuned into the different energies of the family and friends who had left this world. The love I had known with them did not die with their physical selves, it was still there for me when I needed it. Surely then, the affection of those who are still living will follow me too? For Meg, for me, for us all, there is continuity of love across physical distance, as there is across time. If we are not separated from the souls we cherish by the earthly realms, the English Channel shouldn't present me with too much of a problem.

The two older horses were close by. I placed a hand on each of their backs seeking a physical reminder of their strength and calm. 'We are going to live together,' I spoke out loud. A new emotion rose up. I recognised it as relief. And maybe, somewhere, a flicker of excitement.

34

Michael

Letting in

'This will be the last time that we meet here, in this way.' I was sitting opposite Michael, the last of my regular clients to whom I was bidding farewell. He sought support after a spiteful divorce to clear the decks before embarking on a new relationship.

I continued, 'I am aware that there is some regret around for me today as I am preparing for my move. It is important to share that with you. I am sorry that we will not be working together anymore.'

'Well, you never know I might just make it over to France and join one of the retreats you will be doing. You won't get rid of me so easily!' Michael's lightness of tone was welcome.

'What would you like from your time with the herd today?' I asked.

'I will leave that to them, I've been here often enough to know that they will decide what I need.'

The next hour was one of those which felt as spacious as a day while it was happening, but as short as a minute, once it was over. Each moment lived to the full, without reference to the one before or one to come. An onlooker would have seen a man in his late fifties, with a sweatshirt tied by the sleeves around his waist, resting awhile with each of the three horses grazing in the field, before ambling over to the next. Here and there a muzzle lifted, a hand placed on a wither, a back stroked.

A distance away, a woman stood in the shadow of a tree, shifting her weight from time to time. There was no need, today, for intervention from her. An unremarkable scene, yet one which held so much.

'OK, I'm done, I think.' Michael's grin came from inside.

'Looks like you are. Would you like to share anything with me about your experience?' I asked.

'You know, when I arrived I thought it didn't really matter what happened today. I felt I had already got what I needed from our sessions, that it was pretty much done and dusted.'

'And…?'

'When I was out there with those guys again, enjoying being together, everything fell into place. In doing *nothing* this morning I seem to have understood *everything*. Since Mandy and I separated, I have kept my body and my mind so busy, trying to get over it. Maybe, too, wanting to prove that … I don't know … I'm a good person … that someone else will want to be with. I guess I felt tainted by the failure of my marriage and that I'd be 'tarnished goods'. But out there today I realised that letting go of my wife and all that went with our marriage isn't about racking my brains to make sense of it all, or scrabbling around on the internet to find my next partner, or even creating a wall-to-wall social life. Moving forwards isn't about 'letting go' at all. It is about 'letting in'. I was happy this morning for no other reason than I allowed myself to be. I let those good feelings *in*. I was amazed at how effortless it was.'

I tidied the therapy room for the last time reflecting on Michael's wise words. Preparing ourselves for change was not about letting go, it was about *letting in*. I was trying to release my stress, work loose my ties, to help me leave. But I was meeting internal resistance, which was confusing and provoked anxiety. Of course it did. Because I didn't actually *want* to let go of my nurturing life in Wiltshire. And why on earth would I? Yet if I thought about making space to 'let in' the new life I was seeking, and the bounty which it would bring, this felt so much more possible. Imagining that I was making space for newness brought me comfort and enabled me to reach out to those who urged me on towards my new horizon.

PART TWO

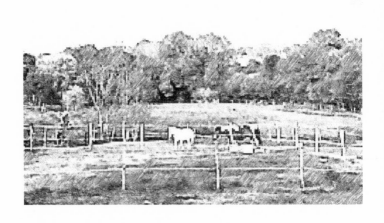

35

Arrival

October 2018

The horses drift together through the ancient grassland. We are separated only by the garden fence. They are happy, looking as if they always lived here. Their tails taken by the breeze dance weightlessly like spiders' threads. My dogs dive from one grassy hummock to the next, sending soil flying beneath them as they dig for elusive field mice. They, too, are in their element.

The final weeks in the UK blurred one into the next. I lived on a knife-edge. What could go wrong did. I cried often and shouted a little. I nearly called the move off several times, but then I would go to the herd, take strength from them and steel myself for the next administrative or emotional peak I had to scale. After three return cross-channel journeys I am here, now, in France for better or worse. There is no going back. I know that I am deeply exhausted.

Behind me is the farmhouse, a place I do not yet like to be, its walls whispering of its previous residents. They seemed to be kind people so I am surprised to feel uncomfortable with the energy which was left. Stacks of cardboard boxes in the centre of every room add to the inhospitable atmosphere. So here, outside on the terrace, I retreat. The unusually kind late autumn affords me an outdoor living space until the dampness of the evening descends.

To my right I look up the valley, the land folding in on itself where small copses offer colourful sprays of gold. To my left, the pasture rolls away on up to an old stone barn which I know will provide shelter on hot summer days. At the boundary of the garden erupts a natural spring. It feeds a small pond which in turn trickles out to the stream at the foot of the valley. My ears are full with its lullaby and the symphony of birdsong all around.

Facing me across the small valley lies a farm. The old buildings in my line of sight are not pretty having been abandoned long ago for modern structures over the crest of the hill. Yet I am at ease with this reminder of what has been. I have chosen to live in the heart of an agricultural community. Farm buildings there must be.

I watch Millie, still a little unsure of herself even after a year with us. She makes a tentative request to step into Ruby's space. She rests her chin on the mane of the blazing chestnut matriarch who tolerates the contact, unusually. It is the first time I have witnessed a relaxation of the boundaries imposed on the younger horse, by which physical contact has previously been denied. Ruby is not yet ready to offer the mutual grooming which Millie wants so she soon drifts away.

In the absence of knowing

I observe these small changes in the herd's behaviour with curiosity. How will our relationships evolve now that we live side by side? Now that I am no longer a visitor what will I become to them, and they to me? They are unruffled after landing in this strange place. I wonder, did they sense the mental images I have been sharing with them of this beautiful destination and the long transit they would take in the lorry?

Using these positive thoughts helped me, if not them, in the days before the move. When the terror felt too much to bear, when my nerves prevented me from sleeping, when I sobbed at my desk asking why I was putting myself through it all, I

130

would hold this picture of us all here, bathed in sunshine, and feel instantly reassured.

My cheeks are cooled by a light breeze. A flock of long-tailed tits swoop in front of me and take up noisy residence in the pear tree nearby. The agony of decision making, searching, planning, implementing and saying goodbye is over. It is pointless now to worry about whether I was right to come. In spite of, or perhaps even because of, my emotional and physical depletion, I am now fully available to soak up the simple pleasure of existing. The future lies open before me. Without any sense of how it will unfold, or how it will be for me to live here, I take unexpected comfort from the uncertainty. In the absence of 'knowing', all that there is left, is to trust.

I would need to remember this if I was to survive what was to come.

36

The Dignity of Choice

November 2018

It would take months to regain my usual levels of effervescence, to gather up the parts of me which had not yet arrived and contain them lovingly back into my body. But winter was facing us and there was much work to be done.

I set about finding good tradesmen and within two weeks of arriving the place was a hive of activity, with dangerous fencing being torn down, the hay barn roof replaced and a small corral with hard-standing in front of the cow-shed constructed. The horses, this year, would be able to stay out of the mud and take shelter in the lee of the barn. Later I would have the cowshed adapted so that they had entry at will. Compared to what they were used to, they would be living in luxury.

Before I knew it a month had passed. It was already early December. Taking a break on the terrace I enjoyed the first day of solitude with no workmen expected. The mild autumn had been gentle on the landscape and golden leaves fluttered against the blue morning sky. It was bliss sitting in this spot where the land wrapped itself around me in a soothing embrace. I felt rooted, close to nature and with a quiet mind.

I watched the horses leaving the corral which lay up the slope to my right. They travelled in single file, nose to tail out into the field which tipped precariously into my small valley. They could almost have been one of those paper chains cut skilfully out of folded paper, so symmetrical was their movement.

With temporary fencing I had set up a track so that they could move around the land without having access to too much grass. Now I observed them travelling along it, passing in front of me, all acknowledging me with a tip of the nose as they passed. Here and there they paused and lingered, nibbling and savouring whatever morsels they found.

A new aura

At the moment that Ruby paused to look at me, the sun emerged above the tree line and illuminated her fiery golden mane, crowning her and the copse beyond in glorious splendour. Moisture embellished each branch with a thousand diamonds each with its own unique light source. Watching the herd dispersing into the adjacent field, I registered an aura to them as they moved. Was it the way in which their coats reflected the sunlight and contrasted with the backdrop of autumnal foliage or had there been some other shift? It took me some time to discern what I was sensing. That was it – they moved now with huge *dignity*.

Horses are embodied naturally with this quality but now it seemed to be enhanced in them. Within what was possible in these five acres of mine, my herd had developed a routine in which they followed the sun and escaped the weather. They knew which spots would be graced with the first and last rays of the day and where to go to escape the prevailing wind. There were corners they liked to sleep, rest and cleanse. It was already some years since any of them had been stabled, but here there seemed to be a difference. Here they had everything that they needed: shelter, shade, fresh water, slopes, wild herbs and overhanging trees to forage. Here, they possessed the dignity which stemmed from choice.

37

Toxic at the Top

I had not paid particular attention to the concept of dignity for a long time. My mind turned to a development intervention I had delivered a few months earlier for the senior management team of a large global corporation. The quality of the experience was polar opposite to the harmonious scene I was witnessing as my herd settled in this tranquil environment. What happened had been troubling me.

The charismatic CEO talked the talk of empowerment, culture change and empathic leadership when my colleague and I met him to take the brief. As the first morning of the event unfolded an allegiance between him and one of the directors slowly manifested. This was the power-base and the rest of the team formed two groups – those who sought their protection through sycophantic behaviour, and those who tried to keep themselves hidden at all costs. In this way no-one was making a real contribution other than at a technical 'toe the line' sort of level.

The truth will out

When contracting with any new client I always emphasise that there is nowhere to hide with the horses. The truth will always out. If teams are not ready or willing to address their difficulties, I advise that it is best not to come to work with us. The counsel went unheeded and what transpired during the workshop was uncomfortable for everyone involved.

The herd responded in their typically honest and direct way. They avoided the two dominant leaders at all costs, flattening ears and swishing tails as they left in a cloud of dust. Those team members who curried favour were gently pushed around by their equine learning partners, and those who tried to stay invisible were ignored. Very quickly blame for the chaos which ensued was attributed unsparingly to the most vulnerable members of the team. And finally on the second day, as the situation deteriorated still further, the horses, and then I and my team, became the fall-guys.

The experience stayed with me for weeks. Aside of being disappointed that I had not been able to help these people, there was something so utterly painful about it all. Every member of the team was dehumanised in some way by those with the power and they all adopted varying types of avoidant behaviour. None were left with their dignity. And none seized it back.

Leading for dignity

Whether we are leading a team, leading ourselves or leading our horses, an important part of that leadership is to preserve dignity without which 'our best' is not possible. At the times when I lost mine, or rather had it taken from me by either small or large injustices, I understood much later how shame took its place. My need to avoid the gut-hollowing feeling that humiliation provokes prevented me from addressing what had happened. Instead, I pretended that it hadn't. It was easier that way. But by doing so I colluded to perpetuate the undignified place to which I was shunted, as some of the members of this Board were doing.

When we find that our self-respect is compromised in this way, it isn't always within our ability to respond. Sometimes we are too vulnerable, too afraid of the consequences. Other times circumstance dictates that it just isn't possible to vote with our feet. Yet the road to recovering our sense of self and our confidence begins at the moment we acknowledge the nature of our experience. The first step to retrieving our dignity is in saying 'Enough!' and we have to say this first to ourselves. Whether coercive behaviour is pursuing us within marriage, a friendship, our family or even in the boardroom where six-figure salaries are the norm.

38

Winter Solstice

December 2018

Whilst the horses had enjoyed an upgrade to their living quarters, I had been relegated to Economy class. Even though the ancient oil-fired boiler roared like a NASA rocket, it didn't heat the house. A string of plumbers came, most ended up sucking their teeth and shaking their heads. Nothing could be done other than install a completely new heating system.

There was a huge wood-burner in the lounge, whose size was conversely proportionate to its efficiency. The paltry heat it created quickly leached from the cracks in the doors, window frames and stone walls. As I pulled my thermals on each morning I thought wistfully of the small, well-insulated home I had left behind and the roaring log-fire which would have welcomed me at the local pub.

Winter Solstice marked the end of a tumultuous year. I knew that according to Eastern practice, I was meant to be reconnecting, focusing on re-birth and re-creation. Yet I felt utterly blue. I missed folks in the UK. There would have been carol singing, festive meals, parties and presents. I'd have been looking forward to the chink of bubbly glasses on Christmas morning followed by a long dog walk before a dinner shared. In France I would be alone on December 25th for the first time in my life. I had not felt so low for a long time.

I turned my attention that evening to preparing myself a delicious, healthy meal. Good food is always guaranteed to cheer me up. I chose a Latin playlist on my i-pad, turned it up to drown out the whirring of the extractor fan and gyrated whilst stirring the simmering pans. Suddenly a loud hissing noise made me spin round. The kitchen radiator, bizarrely placed on the wall *above* the tall American style fridge, had transformed into a geyser. Steaming water erupted from eight feet high. It was then that I realised I knew nothing about central heating systems or even where the stop cock was.

I ran upstairs, grabbed all the towels I could lay my hands on and picked up my phone on the way back. Climbing on a chair I jammed towels around the burst pipework to divert the scalding trajectory. Instead of spraying into the room it ran down the walls instead. I wasn't sure if this was any wiser given the proximity of the nearest power socket. I rang the only person I knew who might be able to help me. He arrived twenty minutes later, turned off the water supply and isolated the radiator in question. I don't remember ever being so pleased to see someone.

By 9.30pm I had still not eaten my meal but I did have a very clean kitchen floor. I went outside to top up the horses' hay for the night, they nickered when they heard me crunching across the gravel. A sound to lift my mood under any circumstances. There, backlit against a cinematographic sky the three of them stood. The invisible moon cast its brilliant light from its hiding place over the horizon, gilding the fluffy clouds which raced away from me as they retreated into the inky blackness. Observing the different layers of this montage, that I had a cold house mattered not. Nor that I was missing the fun of the festive season in England. What could be more uplifting, more giving of meaning, than this, here, right now?

Almost to a cue the moon lifted itself into view. I felt as if I could reach up and touch it with my gloved fingertips. It ducked and dived elusively, shifting shadows and shades of black, grey, silver up and down the monochrome valley.

Gathered with the three horses and two terriers under its magnificent light my regrets dissolved into a deep sense of awe.

39

Christmas

25th December 2018

Millie's mane glowed with an LED brightness reflecting the
first kiss of sunlight. From opal blue to dusky pink the heavens
transformed. Even the ugly farm-buildings shone majestically.
Waking birds bobbed while an owl still hooted. Above the
huge poplar, rooted in the foot of the valley and with great
pompoms of mistletoe, a lone star still beamed. Perhaps it was
the same star which the Three Kings had followed.

Christmas. Contemplating the day ahead without human
company, unexpectedly, I felt no dread. Memories of all the
other Christmas days connected like a long corridor and invited
me to step into it. Rooms decorated with the trees and
handmade decorations of my childhood, tables laden with food
cooked lovingly by my mother, pillowcases stuffed with small
gifts and citrus scented tangerines, the candle which glowed in
the porch to show Santa the way to his biscuits and the carrots
left for the reindeer. Later, on grown-up Christmas days, where
I broke from tradition and cooked a paella, or walked through
the frost before quiet meals around the fire.

There wasn't only happiness. There was that lethal blade,
cutting to a visceral place when all around me were smiling and
I felt only grief. Yet, when all my lived days connected, a wave
of love reached towards me.

Just because today I would be alone, did not mean that I
had to be lonely. The air above my head was displaced by a

140

swooping flock of chaffinches. I erupted into spontaneous laughter. I was, absurdly, outrageously happy. I felt connected with those pieces of me which I had shared with others both past and presently and which they held in their hearts, and the parts of them which I cherished in mine.

I remembered the feeling of being alongside Zeus, the feral pony from the moors. How I felt, through him, time open up simultaneously rather than being a string of sequential events. Now, beside Millie, this feeling settled into my core. I was beginning to understand the edges of what this meant and that it brought me everything I needed.

None of the love or laughter of my life lived before was lost. The pain of loss, at its most acute on this day of the year, had not vanished either. Yet I was strong enough now to hold it in balance with compassion and care. I could be with it peacefully.

40

Exploring the Corners of Solitude

January 2019

They left a wake of laughter and love behind them. I waved at the head of the driveway for longer than they could see me: my late brother's widow, Kate, her husband and my two nephews, now grown into young, tall and equally handsome men. Several years after Gordon passed away, Kate, my sister-in-spirit remarried. Two bereaved families were joined whilst honouring those they lost.

I surveyed the living room where we spent the cold evenings between Christmas and New Year, playing cards, board games, chatting and being easy with each other. My nephews, strikingly like their father, brought joyful memories of him and revived in me a sense of generational belonging which had slipped away. My remaining younger brother had lived in the French Alps for over twenty years and we seldom saw each other.

The house felt more like home after my visitors. Now that they had gone it seemed so quiet. Throwing on a coat, I took my morning drink into the garden. I felt out of sorts. I needed to adjust to the solitude, within which dwelled melancholy, but also, I acknowledged with interest, a hint of relief.

I contemplated the six winter weeks which lay, blandly, before me. There were no other guests expected nor social events planned. My next work engagement was in mid-February when I would travel back to the UK for the first time to deliver a client leadership development programme. It risked being a bleak intervening period.

Who knows what you might find in solitude?

The last time that I stepped away from the life I knew, although somewhat less dramatically, I went to Colorado to spend six weeks on a ranch learning about horsemanship. I came back, not a different person, but so much closer to the one I was meant to be. Within a year I changed my life beyond recognition.

And here I was again, embarking on a great adventure alone. It was gutsy, some said crazy. Yet in the corners of my alone-ness what might I find? Perhaps even more of myself than I had discovered before.

My spirits lifted immeasurably. An excitement brewed at this blank page which lay in front of me. I had thrown my doors wide open to possibility. Far from feeling daunted by the solitude, the strength which comes from grasping change was taking up residence in my bones. It was for me to make of my life here what I chose.

41

The Nail

Winter revealed its ugly side. Relentlessly heavy rain blew horizontally up the valley for days. The horses wore their winter rugs and found shelter in the lee of the hay barn where they waited in an eager line for me each morning. So, when I slid the barn doors open and saw Winston immobile at the far end of the corral, in the full force of the weather, my stomach lurched. He held one front leg off the ground and carried tension around his eyes and muzzle.

I put the buckets down for the other two and hurried to his side. Lifting the foot, I saw a bent nail embedded in the sole protruding by over an inch. I touched it gently with a finger but he flinched and reared on his good leg. Quickly I tied Ruby and Millie out of the way before reaching for my phone.

Call in vain

It was still early and there was no answer from my farrier. I called the vet. His receptionist rang me back two minutes later. 'I'm sorry he is busy,' she announced. 'You will have to bring the horse here to the clinic this afternoon in your lorry. He can see you then.'

I was in rural France. There were only two vets covering a large region. It wasn't like the UK where any one of several local practices could have had someone with me in fifteen minutes. I thought of ringing my English farrier or vet for advice but with the time difference they were probably not even awake.

Winnie was getting tired of standing. Every time he tried to put his foot down it was clearly agony. There was no way he could walk, never mind get in a lorry. And any pressure on his foot would just drive the nail deeper. It sank in with a sick feeling that I would have to deal with this myself.

I rushed around grabbing what I would need: pliers to pull the nail, antiseptic to clean the foot, salt water in a bucket in which to clean it, then everything I would need to dress the foot - poultice, bandage, plastic for a waterproof wrapping, scissors, tape, anything else? I ticked each item off in my head.

The rain lashed down and the spot where Winnie was standing was under an inch of water. I couldn't move him so I would have to get it all done without him putting his foot down if I was to avoid any further chance of infection.

'OK my love. We can do this.' I laid my hand on his neck as I spoke and looked him in the eye. I pictured what would happen and imagined it going well, soothing myself as I did. 'You are going to be OK. But it might hurt. OK big fella. Let's do this.'

I took Winston's foot and gently grasped the nail with the pliers as close to the sole as I could. He flinched, snatching back his hoof. I broke into a sweat, my mouth dry. Should I be doing this at all? I didn't know, but what options did I have?

He allowed me to try again, but reared this time. How I longed to be back in England waiting for professional help that I could rely on. Why the hell had I come to this god-forsaken place? Choking down my escalating concern, wiping the blinding rain from my face, I closed my eyes and breathed deeply. 'Stay with me, Winnie. Let me help you. I don't know what else I can do.'

He touched me with his muzzle. This felt like permission. The pliers gripped the nail and I exerted every ounce of strength. It moved a fraction and although a jolt of pain shot

145

through him he kept his other three feet on the ground long enough for me to take the strain again. The nail slid out bringing with it a spurt of blood. Thank God. I lathered his foot clean with disinfectant, before plunging it into the bucket of salt water. He blew out, his sides heaving as he released long held breath. He rested his nose in my cupped hands, motionless, grateful, relieved.

The worst was done, but there was work still to do before I could succumb to the shake which had started in my knees. He seemed to know how important it was to keep his foot up and out of the dirty puddle until the wound was dressed and waterproofed with several layers of plastic and tape. My arms went around his neck, my emotion flooded into his long damp mane. He curled his neck about me, placing the lightest of contact with his cheek on the small of my back as if in a hug.

Something special happened between us. I wasn't sure exactly what it was.

42

Lunar Halo

Reality sinks in

Winston recovered from his injury quickly. The first month of the year slipped by with rain turning to sleet, then snow and fog with ice. There was even a freezing rain which coated the world in fine slippery glass making it impossible to leave the house for several days.

I battled paperwork as I was bounced around the region by French bureaucrats in my attempts to register my car, my residence, and my business. Even buying insurance here required a two-hour meeting at the bank or agency. Two such meetings ended after an afternoon of form-filling to be told that for incomprehensible reasons my vehicles and I were currently uninsurable. The concept of patience was taking on a completely new meaning.

My mood flipped from exasperated, to confused, to bewildered. The house was cold, the nights long and dark. Wintertime here didn't seem to offer much joy. Being so badly supported at a veterinary level had rattled me. After only two months it felt like my honeymoon with this life I had chosen may be over.

My tonic

One night, with six degrees below freezing, I wrapped my snug coat around me. Poppy, my devoted Jack Russell, scurried to my side at the sound of my hand on the door and scampered ahead of me up to the barn. Given her tiny frame, it was strange to find her presence so reassuring. Ostensibly I braved the dark nights in order to top up the hay supply, but the act was more for me than the horses. However frustrating my day had been time cocooned with the herd put me right. I could later brave the glacial bedroom feeling that, in the end, it would all be worthwhile.

The moonlight bounced off the stone walls of the farmhouse throwing eerie shadows across the path. Unusually bright, even for a full moon. I glanced upwards and there it was, hanging high, held within a great circle of white light which spread its reach across the entire valley. I had never seen anything like it, a divine bullseye of utter brilliance, blotting out even the brightest of stars. Three steely forms in the pasture nickered when they sensed me and approached like phantoms. I stayed a long while with them that night, entranced by the magnificence in the sky.

Choosing experience

The next day I discovered that I had witnessed a lunar halo. The phenomenon is caused when the light of the moon is refracted through ice crystals in the atmosphere. Like a rainbow, a lunar halo can be made of any primary colours and its manifestation is situational. If I had not been where I was, when I was, I would not have seen it. What an extraordinary gift it had been. The following night a second halo appeared, this time it was smaller and tinged with pink and soft green, bathing the land in a more gentle glow.

These extraordinary planetary offerings were available to me because I had been there to receive them. I wouldn't have seen them anywhere else. I'd have other experiences here, too, specific to my circumstances. Both good and bad. How easily I allowed recent setbacks to slide me into a negative frame of

148

mind. Were they not part and parcel of my experience? Was this not what living a full life was about? No-one ever said that living your dream was easy, or indeed should be. More than ever I was reminded that the quality of my life experience is dictated by how I choose to see it, and indeed whether I am present and available in the moment to 'see' it at all.

43

Participating

February 2019

Over the years I had invested significantly in learning to 'pay attention'. The success of my work depended on it, my personal health practices involved it. Yet here I was, emerging from behind a fine screen of negativity which lingered between me and appreciation of my new world. Change had swallowed me up and driven me inward. From there I had been peeping cautiously out through a narrow crack in the door.

The invitation

It had been sitting on my table since before Christmas. An A4 notice announcing a 'Cérémonie des Fêtes' at the commune's Mairie on a Saturday morning at 11am. I learned from my neighbours that this was a biannual gathering of citizens where the mayor of the parish would share the council's plans for the year, discuss the budget and explain spending in the previous period. It sounded uninteresting to say the least.

The day arrived. Shyness, coupled with a reluctance to remove any of the toasty clothing I wore to put on something smarter, dissuaded me from attending. I made a hot drink and began to settle myself for a day indoors. The dazzling image of the lunar halo and its teaching appeared in my mind. I needed to show up, to this event and others. I had to be available if I was to receive.

150

With only fifteen minutes to go before the meeting began, I retained my thermals but swapped my fleece and jeans for a sweater dress, grabbed my car keys and shot out of the door. Time in the French countryside operates on a different plane and I should not have fretted about being late. I was one of the first to arrive. As I locked my car a whole stream of vehicles began to arrive behind me and were abandoned untidily on the verges.

Inside the large village hall a number of trestle tables formed an island in the centre of the space. Immaculate tablecloths, clearly donated by different households, created a patchwork muddle of colours and fabrics. I stood amidst the hand-shaking, cheek-kissing locals wishing I had not come. Everyone appeared to know each other so well. Then suddenly my hand was being grasped, my arm shaken almost out of my shoulder socket and the first introduction made.

There were no signs of a speech from the mayor, but trays of sparkling wine and small snacks were being passed around. This was perhaps the earliest lunchtime aperitif I had ever had. Before very long I was the person whom everyone wanted to meet and, to my horror, kiss. Elderly ladies whose whiskers shared the crisps they had just eaten with me, stooping farmers who left a trail of spittle on my cheek, teenagers who wanted to practice their English and small children who stared in fascination at the stranger in their midst. I found a handful of women with whom small talk was easier, and from there I was hosted and hailed.

I noticed in particular how kind people were with each other. Those who were infirm or unable to stand were courted at their seats and wheelchairs. Toddlers were adored, spouses flirted and not always with each other. To my surprise I was actually having fun.

It was a long cry from the fashionable Saturday morning breakfast I might have had before in my favourite canal-side cafe. But these people were now my neighbours and I could not have been more delighted to meet them.

44

Margaret's Story

The hills around the farm rolled back, blanched fields relaxing under a February sun. I was back in Wiltshire to deliver the first client interventions of the year, of which there would be two that month. After a period of relatively isolated living, finding myself on the English motorways rammed with traffic and angry people, had been destabilising. Here, with my feet on the turf, surrounded by my colleagues, our clients and the grounding presence of the horses I was coming back into my body.

When it transpired that I would be supporting the small group allocated to Juniper and his herd mate Tommy I couldn't help but feel pleased. The exquisitely elegant ex-racehorse had touched me deeply during our last work together when he coaxed Dwight, a reserved, private man out of his shell. Juniper carried in his eye the sadness of a soul which was once broken, the brilliance of one which had healed, and the softness of a spirit which he now generously shared with us.

Sorting the men from the boys

Margaret crossed the paddock in efficient strides and landed squarely in front of Tommy, a great docile hunk of a horse, with ears as long as his head was wide.

'You look like you mean business,' she boomed and slapped him on the shoulder. His part-Shire muscle rippled under the force of her contact. He carried on grazing, showing moderate disdain with a small flick of his voluminous tail. I quietly reminded Margaret that it is important to wait for the horses to initiate physical contact. She nodded, harrumphed and began to circle him, rubbing her chin in problem-solving mode.

I was surprised when Juniper sidled quietly up to Margaret, head slightly lowered and muzzle extended in greeting. She looked straight through him as if he wasn't there and moved around to the other side of Tommy. The graceful racer lifted his head, fixing her with a lengthy gaze, then stretched his neck down to eat.

A senior vice-president in the company she worked for, Margaret had outlined a desire to improve the dynamism of her management team at the start of the day. 'This year's results are crucial. I need them at the top of their game. At the moment they are not.' Her tone was perfunctory.

'What do you need them to do differently?' I asked.

'Our organisation is set for a rapid period of growth, but frankly my team are not up to it. They don't drive delivery in their business units. It isn't enough anymore to be good technically, they need to start shaking people up, sorting out the men from the boys.'

Her choice of phrase had piqued my curiosity, as did her rejection of Juniper.

The glass ceiling

Margaret was now in dogged pursuit of Tommy who was ignoring her, as she had done to his field-mate. The furrows on her brow deepened. The coaching I offered was batted away with the wave of a hand. The session ended and an angry silence followed her back to the rest of the group.

I felt for Margaret as she witnessed one after the other of her peers gel affectionately with both of the willing geldings.

Given the success of the rest of the group, we progressed after lunch to a phase of haltering and walking alongside our learning partners. Tommy, the most genial and gentle giant, moved not a muscle for Margaret. Every time she reached to clip the rope onto his headcollar his soft lashes blinked benignly before turning his huge nose away from her without so much as moving a toe. She bustled from one side of him to the other, following his movement.

'Perhaps we could take time out and have a walk around the paddock Margaret,' I suggested. She stepped in beside me and we ambled to the furthest corner of the field.

'How is this experience for you right now?' I asked.

'Excruciating, humiliating, defeating. It is the worst day I can remember in my business career to date.'

'And ... what else?'

'What else is there?' Margaret barked. 'I have failed in front of my colleagues, who have all succeeded. You can't imagine or understand how that is for me.'

'Try me.'

Her anger boiled over. 'I've worked tirelessly in this organisation to succeed at the highest level, to break through the wretched glass ceiling which no-one will ever acknowledge. I have farmed out childcare, given up so much of my family life. Everyone looked up to me and now – I must be a laughing stock.'

There was an aliveness to one phrase, which I wanted to pursue. 'Is there anything else which you have given up Margaret?'

A long pause, then with a deep sigh her resentment collapsed and she sounded suddenly weary.

'I guess I have given up myself. Given up *on* myself too. You can only get to the top in this business world, you know, by being more of a man than a man. It is the price a woman has to pay. I am tired of it.'

155

I recalled the early days of my own career spent in the manufacturing industry and the struggle it had often been. How I had developed a thick skin during that time. Eventually I had opted out, first joining an organisation where I was valued, and later working for myself. Margaret had however continued to carry the gauntlet. It was thus with great empathy that I continued.

'I wonder whether the personal authority which you have embodied over the years belongs to *you* Margaret - or if it belongs to the person you feel that others expect you to be? Can you close your eyes and get a sense of that? Get in touch with what *you* stand for, and feel it right down to your feet.'

Succeeding because of

The woman closed her eyes, tipped back her head and her chest lifted with an intake of fresh air.

'It's hard to tell the difference, to be honest. My sense of myself has got so mixed up with the role I feel I need to play. But I can say that what I value is fairness and I suppose that is why I have fought so hard to have the success I know I deserve.'

I nodded and continued. 'Your innate qualities will command even more respect Margaret than the ones you have been borrowing, because they are stronger. When you allow them to be fully seen, you will succeed *because of* your gender and not *in spite of* it. That would be so valuable for all the women you are leading to see.'

Margaret's expression made me wonder if I had gone too far. We walked in silence back to where Tommy and Juniper were grazing.

'What shall I do now, then?' she asked contritely.

'Let them decide that. See what they have to offer you.'

I was sure that she would be safe on her own with these two kindest of creatures, so stood in the shade of the oak tree

156

where Margaret's colleagues waited. I watched the huge mass that was Tommy cross the ten feet of turf one hoof at a time. The woman reached up a hand and stroked his nose. Juniper joined them and the three rested. After a matter of minutes, both horses let out a discreet sigh and the movement of their sides indicated they were breathing slower and deeper. Something was changing for Margaret in her inner world.

Day Two came. Margaret was pale and her sharpness had gone. She no longer dominated conversations and made only one request for the day, that she could work again with Tommy and Juniper.

'I'm going to let what happens happen. They gave me so much food for thought – I am used to driving, pushing, controlling. Leadership feels like a daily battle to be won. I approached the horses in the same way yesterday. It's no wonder that Tommy didn't want anything to do with me. I've been reflecting on how it must be for my team. How many times have I alienated them by not acknowledging their presence or their willingness to try things, like I did with Juniper? Or how many times do they disengage because I am only interested in what they produce. So ...today ... well I am going to do as you say and try to lead from an authentic place. Be like the person I am at home, where I am so different.'

The day which followed was a caring and happy one for the group of four to which Margaret belonged. The vulnerability she had embraced invited others to do the same. Their learning partners responded with kind cooperation. Juniper revealed more of himself too, as she did. He became playful, his slender legs growing long and his movement balletic as he walked and trotted around the field.

When we closed the programme, china plates piled with cake and mugs brimming with tea, Margaret, her eyes sparkling and complexion rosy, spoke first.

'I need to talk to you all about something which is important both for me at a personal level, and also for us all as leaders in our business.' She spoke with firm calmness, her vocal chords mellow where before they had been strained. 'Most of you here are men, and please don't take offence because what I am about to say is not about you as individuals or really even you as a collective, it is about our culture. For a woman to succeed she has to be even more of a 'man' than a man. The dynamic is well-known in our society and yet it barely changes for all the policies we have put in place and statistics which we bandy around. Our culture puts pressure on young women coming up our ranks to betray the very qualities which we need them for. We have seen it today with the horses. We didn't get the best from them, and we don't from our people, by pushing them beyond their limits, controlling them or criticising them. But when we relate to them with compassion and kindness, and we try to understand them, anything is possible. Like it or not, these feminine qualities, possessed by both males and females of course, are eroded in our organisation's culture.'

Recognition and acknowledgement rippled around the room. The other two women present declared 'Hear, Hear!'

'What support would you like from your colleagues Margaret, to make the personal changes which you would like to embrace?' I asked.

She looked around the room, taking gentle eye contact with each of her colleagues, all peers in different parts of the business.

'It is going to feel awkward for me, and perhaps for others too, as I try to behave differently. Feedback would be good. And encouragement. When I get back to work next week I will start by getting together with each of my management team to talk about where they are at and what they need from me. Perhaps the chance to talk over what I learn from them with someone from this group would be a good idea?'

Margaret's tentative suggestion was popular and everyone quickly organised themselves into 'buddy' pairs who would

158

support each other when they got back to the workplace. The programme drew to a satisfying close and there was a particularly strong sense of completeness for me as my co-facilitators and I hugged our farewells.

45

Where is Home?

Just a matter of months separated me from the life I had known in Wiltshire. After my work was concluded I stayed on for a few days crammed with laughter, chatter, coffees, teas, meals out and walks in the winter sun. It felt good to be back. My psyche tricked me into believing that I might walk through my old front door to an enthusiastic greeting from my dogs, put the kettle on and throw myself into my favourite chair in the sunny conservatory. I was greeted in the local cafes and the village pub affectionately with exclamations of 'You look so well! French life is suiting you!'

What I felt on the inside was not entirely showing. As I shunted from one wonderful reunion to another, I kept thinking 'I left all this ... all this ... LOVE.' A part of me looked on at what I had done, aghast. And yet neither could I deny that my new lifestyle was clearly good for me. I was caught between my two worlds.

After a weekend socialising it was time to return to France. At the ferry terminal the night was dark and my spirits went into free-fall. The hour until embarkation, when I could slide into my bunk and await the oblivion of sleep, stretched unsympathetically before me. Tilting my car seat back I closed my eyes and let my thoughts flit across the glad images, feelings and sensations of the past week.

'I gave up all that.' The words hit me like a sledgehammer.

Integrating change

My mind turned to Margaret and what she had shared with me. How she had sacrificed much of herself to succeed at work, and by doing this had become rigid and sharp. I posed myself the same question I had offered to her just a few days earlier. What had I sacrificed to go to France? I began to create an inventory – it was more of a series of images than a list – of people, places, habits, vistas - of everything which I loved about my 'old' life. As I made space for these feelings, their impact softened. I was able to show myself kindness and understanding.

I probed deeper like I had with Margaret. What else had I given up? This time the images which came to me were altogether less pleasant: struggling to cope in the mid of winter, crying with frustration, fingers hurting from the cold and unable to stay upright in the sludge; lying in bed worrying about the ponies when they were sick and I couldn't get to check on them; the hay wagon getting stuck or having to dig my way through the snow with containers of water.

I made a quiet space around my next question, 'What have I gained?' The reply came in a fanfare. I could see the horses from anywhere in my garden, see them at any minute of every day. I had moved to a beautiful country I loved for heaven's sake. Beyond that – I had to accept that I didn't know what else I would be gaining by starting this new life. It was too early to know. But I was beginning to integrate the enormity of the transition I had made. The emotional, physical and spiritual impact, the shifting relationships, what I missed as well as what I celebrated.

The glare of headlights from the vehicle behind caused me to open my eyes as the great iron gates rolled back and fluorescent figures emerged to guide us through passport control onto the quay. As I drove up the ramp into the belly of the boat, I knew that home wasn't where I had come from, or

161

even where I was heading. Home was not made of bricks and mortar, it was the place inside me where I belonged to myself.

46

Striving, Wanting and Having

March 2019

When Millie arrived with me over a year earlier I soon discovered that her friendly, curious personality was masked by an intransigent mistrust of human intention. I hoped she would eventually become a pony with whom I could have ridden outings, but at the beginning she only knew how to fight me. I would give her as long as she needed before any retraining began.

It hadn't been difficult to give her that time. There was the winter from hell, followed by multiple house-hunting trips, the property purchase and the relocation process to occupy me. I hadn't been grounded enough to contemplate riding even Ruby, my experienced, long term saddle partner, never mind work with a young horse.

Now as the shy snowdrops under the great lime tree hinted at spring, it felt time to start a more focused conversation with Millie. I wanted to convince her that she could communicate politely and be heard, instead of resisting me with 450kg of muscle and double that of attitude.

Seeking softness

Each morning I set aside half an hour to work with her, always on the ground, following classical training techniques which coax the horse to soften, shape and move in harmony with the

163

handler. Until she felt able to accept the most gentle leadership from me, yielding willingly to requests made, I would not consider so much as sitting on her back. At the outset her physical and emotional bodies were set like stone. When I gently asked her to back away from me, her feet rooted into the ground like the huge oak trees behind us. I didn't take it personally, she behaved the same with Winston and Ruby. They usually resorted to their teeth or hooves to move her and she bore the scars on her body to show for it. I wanted to teach her that things could be different for the two of us. That softness could feel good.

One day after the next brought small successes and soon, when I asked her to tilt her head towards or away from me, she began to offer the tiniest of bend instead of unrelenting brace. But after a few weeks we seemed to reach a plateau. I paused our sessions for a week or so, but Millie was no more enthusiastic once we resumed.

It was time for me to reflect on what was happening between us.

Out in my thinking space in the garden, I opened my journal to see where the pen would take me.

Closing my eyes, first I settled into my chair, tuning into the sounds around me – the birdsongs, the distant hum of a vehicle, the trickling of the brook nearby. How was I, right now? What was I noticing in my body? What thoughts were running through my mind? I scanned from my toes to my crown checking in, looking for signs, making sure that I was fully present.

At first all seemed well. I felt good, calm, alive. Yet my thoughts persistently drew my attention to the house, namely into my office. This was my clue and I began to write.

Old patterns die hard

Since I returned from my business trip to the UK, I had thrown myself into developing the French side of my work – setting dates for retreats and workshops, updating my website, sourcing caterers, planning the landscaping which would be needed, preparing the accommodation, even buying linen and bedding. Amongst all this I allocated some time to spend with Millie. Some time when it suited me, not necessarily her. Progressing my rapport with her was another job on my list. Was I present with her? Probably not.

I had effectively recreated the kind of schedule and lifestyle I moved away from. My subconscious had resorted to a default setting which was hard to shake off. I was *striving*. Why? And for what?

Since a disastrous marriage in my thirties there were not many corners of my psyche that I had not explored during my personal development process. I had arrived at an understanding that my drive to work hard was rooted in the need to please people and win approval. As self-awareness tamed those hungers, pushing myself became about moving towards what I loved doing and felt to be my purpose: creating a business, evolving my horse-led psychotherapeutic and learning approach, publishing for the first time. Now what on earth was the striving all about?

I flicked back to the start of the notebook in my lap. I found what I read a little shocking. The early pages were written seven months earlier as relocation was approaching. My words were steeped in the deepest anxiety and I acknowledged that since then, there had not been any real time to pause. And here I was piling more pressure onto myself again.

165

Loving myself

Why was I again finding it hard to shake free of this pattern of striving? Of wanting something different? Perhaps, I wondered, it was easier 'to want' than 'to have'. Was wanting a habit attached to a belief of not being enough and not having enough? Whereas to enjoy a contented place of 'having' requires acceptance that I *am* enough, and that I *have* enough? Was this the trap I was falling into? I was driving myself to accomplish future goals based on an idea of an alternative state of perfection. But *right now* could be, indeed was, perfection itself. This, I realised, was what loving myself was all about.

I lifted my eyes from the page and looked across to Millie across the fence, her round belly stretched full with hay, comically two tone with mud caking the left side of her body, the right side still shining white.

'OK I get it!' I called across to her. Somewhere in my intention towards her, this sense of inadequacy had got mixed up. I was trying to create an ideal between us rather than being with what was. It wasn't that I should stop trying to teach her a more responsive and cooperative way of being with me. But I realised that I needed to approach my interactions with her without any sense of either of us being lacking. Wholly in a spirit of curiosity to listen to what she had to say and compassion for us both as we sought to find harmony together.

I was enough. She was enough. The journey was about how we connected, not how we performed.

47

Interconnection, Love and Leadership

April 2019

The days lengthened and my first springtime in France erupted. It was a feast for the senses: swathes of colour renewing weekly in the hedgerows, a plethora of birds and insects, red squirrels, hedgehogs, buzzards, herons, coypu (river rodents resembling small beavers) and deer with their young, were all regular visitors on or adjacent to my land. Occasionally even wild boar passed by, the speed of their passage impressive given their bulk and relatively short legs. I was always glad that there was a hedge or stream between us.

Letting go of any residual achievement drive became easy. Sitting still in my garden or loitering amongst the herd no longer felt a luxury but a necessity. If I didn't turn up to this party which the valley was throwing for me, with my eyes open and ready to see, it would pass me by as fast as the itinerant boar. Witnessing the magic of it all seemed important.

I noticed how much more available I was. The horses showed their approval. That they ran to me when I called them was not unusual, but it was the speed and attitude with which they now came which was different – galloping uphill to slide to a halt before me.

Often when I sat meditating or sipping from a steaming mug in my hand one or other of them would meander over, lying down to rest, or dozing as they stood in that gravity-defying way which they do. As I felt more connected to the world around me my sense of 'oneness' with them was strengthening. This, I was realising, was what uprooting myself from England had been about. To know more often and more deeply this sense of contentment and of interconnection with all that is.

Nature's power source

A short time later, I was back in the UK to deliver a leadership programme to a favourite client company whom we worked with regularly. I left all the animals in the care of a good friend I had made in France who lived just a few miles away. Back on Wiltshire soil, I was still carrying this golden nugget of insight with me. It felt a little like a secret long-life battery, plugged into my personal power source. Surrounded by the rolling English landscape with red kites arcing overhead it was not difficult to remain in tune with nature.

The group arrived in the small classroom filled with the scent of fresh coffee, tea and home-made biscuits. There was excitement, openness and warmth. I had a sense that the moments ahead would be good. As we were carried through the two days on a dynamic tide of learning led by the horses I was aware of the much stronger sense of interconnectedness which I was holding. At a subtle but significant level it changed the experience of leadership for me.

Co-creation of experience

Whilst my name and signature were still those on the contract, and I designed the structure of the workshop and gathered the team to deliver it, this was not my show. Within the framework of these two days we were all connected – me, my colleagues and the participants, with the herd in the field, the birds in the sky, the trees offering us shade and shelter, the ancient hills around us, even the invisible deer in the woods at the perimeter of the land. How we all moved through the experience would be co-created. One could not act without affecting the other, an emotion here would be felt there, a word or thought from one would ripple its energy to the next. We were all conjoined, all parts of the same picture, all being held and all holding, influenced by and influencing, all that surrounded us.

With our interconnection held consciously in the forefront of my awareness, I noticed how much easier my role became as the leader of the thirty-five humans and fifteen horses involved in this learning experience. I had for many years, almost always, enjoyed this work I did and it was fair to say that most times our clients departed happy. Yet there had always been a background anxiety, a need 'to get it right', to 'do well', which I had to manage. But here I was now, feeling as if I was floating through the event on the waves of what was meant to be, seeing all, feeling all, with none of that burden, or distraction, which I had previously experienced.

A new kind of leadership

The final afternoon came and it was time for the participants to bear witness to each other. The simplicity of what was demonstrated from one group to the next belied the depth of the transformation. One group groomed the horses and stood by them peacefully while they grazed. Another sat, available for their equine partners to join them which they did, leaning muzzles down to ruffle hair on the top of the human heads. Another foursome led their equine learning partners with a fine piece of string and then no rope at all, as if attached by some invisible glue. There was an exquisiteness to the quality of understanding which these people had created with their horses, each other and ourselves. Uncharacteristic of the environment in which these men and women worked, but so graceful and natural it seemed like their birthright. There was joy, delight, gratitude.

169

This indeed was a new kind of leadership. For me most certainly and I believe also for those I worked with that day. One based on interconnectedness, on relationship, on love. If we embodied this sense, acted with this guidance, how different the world could be. I did not know, then, how we would need these lessons later on.

48

The Angry Gardener

April 2019

The thirty-foot hedges provided less of a windbreak and more of a fortress around two of the four properties making up my hamlet. My fellow residents were locked in a smouldering dislike for each other twenty years old: an elderly couple on one side of the lane, farmers born and raised in this tiny scattering of dwellings, with retired Parisians who previously worked in the media, on the other. The neighbours had not spoken for two decades and ensured that they never had to set eyes on each other by growing the gargantuan evergreen screens. The fourth household, an amiable working Anglo-French couple held the neutral ground.

Neighbours

The farmers had been friendly towards me since my arrival and regularly invited me in for coffee and somewhat one-sided conversation. I struggled to understand the patois they spoke and simply nodded, smiled or wrinkled a brow from time to time, hoping that my facial expression was congruous with the events they were describing. They warned me that the Parisians 'hated the English' and advised me to stay away. Taking it all with a large pinch of salt, I attributed little weight to the stories and determinedly waved to the former TV producer every time I saw him working outdoors in the garden. Time and time again he turned his back on me and presented what felt like a cold shoulder. Perhaps I really wasn't welcome. So, I had postponed the neighbourly visit I would normally have made, for a week, a month, then several.

Today, as I passed on my way back from the market there he was again, weeding the frontage of his drive. I slowed down and waved. He looked up, squinted at me and continued with his work. I get the message, I thought, and drove on through my gates.

Unwelcome energy

Later that morning I was tending the garden when suddenly the herd startled. Their heads shot up, ears alert, eyes fixed unblinking. What on earth was it? Moments later a tall, broad man with dense beard and hair pulled back into an untidy ponytail, swaggered round the corner of the barn, hands on hips. I had forgotten that I had booked a gardener to help me tame the increasingly wild outdoor spaces.

'My strimmers are broken,' he announced, 'so I will start with the lawn this morning, then next week I will do the strimming.'

'Oh,' I said, 'I don't really need you to do the lawn, I have a ride-on mower. It is the harder work which I need help with.'

'Well, today I will have to do the lawns. I've come a long way and I only have my mower with me. Where do you want me to start?'

I was so taken aback that the protests I would have liked to make, that this was not a service I needed or wanted to pay for and that I didn't like his manner either, died quietly in my throat.

'OK,' I said, 'Start at the top up there and work your way down.'

'Shall I throw the cuttings to the horses?'

172

'No, no, please don't! Absolutely not! Cut grass can kill them.' I pointed to the bottom of the sloping lawn where the compost heap was situated.

'What? I have to take it all the way down there?'

'Yes, I am afraid you do.'

He disappeared grumbling under his breath and I heard his garden tractor clatter down the ramp of his trailer. I did not rely on him to comply with my instructions regarding the grass cuttings so hovered with my trowel and secateurs.

Ten minutes later a blood curling scream echoed around the valley followed by the most colourful, lesson in French swear words I had ever had. His curses bounced off the farm buildings a quarter of a mile away. Anxious that he was hurt, I ran up the garden, winding myself in the process. I found him throwing his whole weight against the ride-on mower as he tried to push it out of the soft ground which one of the wheels was whisking into powder.

'Are you OK?' I asked, concerned. He glared at me with a smouldering disdain.

The next hour and a half was peppered with increasingly excessive demonstrations of anger at the slightest provocation, such as the engine stalling, the clippings bag filling too quickly or the sun being too hot. Several times he attacked the machine itself with steel-toed boot. Despite the resemblance to an episode of a well-known English 1970s farce featuring an eccentric hotelier, his Mini and a large tree branch which those of my generation may remember, it was too unnerving to be comical.

The horses and I retreated further and further from this thunderstorm of a man, and the tranquil energy of our haven shrunk from the malevolence rippling around him.

'What time would you like me to come next week?' he barked as he loaded up at the end of his visit.

'The same time, that would be fine.' I lied, as I gave him his money. I felt sufficiently concerned for my own safety not to tackle the subject of his behaviour directly.

Danger of assumption

For the first time since I arrived in France I went to lock the main entrance that evening. In this region front doors were normally left unlocked and car keys often dangled in the ignition. But the intimidating behaviour of my visitor made me uneasy. As the gates clanked shut a red squirrel streaked past me with my two terriers in close pursuit, all disappearing behind the colossal pine fortress into the Parisiens' gardens.

Some minutes later from behind the conifers a woman's voice responded to my hushed and ineffective commands to the canines. 'They are in here, they are fine! Come in to get them!' Two smiling, almost elderly people greeted me. The terriers looked at ease and I suspected that cake might have been shared. 'I'm Christian' the husband lifted a hand towards me, 'and this is my wife, Claudine. You must forgive me, I am pretty much blind these days and can't really see where you are.'

I grasped his palm with both hands. How wrong could I have been and how ready to assume?

A beverage was shared as was the local custom, and on returning home, with a dog under each arm, I removed the chain and padlock from the wrought iron gates. Perhaps the gardener, too, had a story to tell. Even so, later that week I sent a polite text telling him that I wouldn't be needing any further help, and broadcast with it unspoken good wishes.

49

The First Ride

April 2019

Unlike horses, who only need to learn things the once, humans need to be reminded again and again of the lessons which keep us centred, healthy and balanced. In spite of all that I knew, my heart banged noisily against my ribs and my mouth was dry the morning I saddled Ruby up late in April. I had not ridden her for seven or perhaps eight months. I imagined everything that could go wrong and remembered how lacking in confidence my mare usually was when riding out somewhere new. I felt sure that we would not get very far.

A whisper of a breeze ruffled her wispy mane. I stood beside her, scanning my body for the fear which I felt struggling for influence. I closed my eyes and breathed out the tension from my muscles. When my pulse began slowing I positioned myself on the mounting block and Ruby sidestepped towards me. She was ready, perhaps more so than I.

Out on the lane, scents rose from the verges and their rainbow of violas, fuchsia-pink orchids, clumps of fragrant lemon balm, daisies and cowslips with their delicate yellow bell-like blooms. Ruby suddenly hesitated, losing confidence.

Harmony rediscovered

'Come on, I will walk with you for a while.' I jumped down and we continued side by side. When her stride started to lengthen beyond my pace I asked her to stop and swung myself back into the saddle. From there, with a loose rein and a song we made our way. I felt the joy which comes from contactful exchange with a horse who sees into my soul. Our route had not been exciting, our speed far from exhilarating, but the thrill of this rediscovered harmony went to my very core.

The dust flew in a great cloud around her as Ruby rolled then shook herself down, a sweaty saddle shaped patch on her back. Leaving the tending of the veg bed for another day, I opened up the sunshade and observed the herd quietly from the garden.

The infinity of right now

Hours slid by effortlessly, time losing its meaning in the infinite moment that 'right now' became. I reflected on how different our outing was to that which I expected. There was no sign of the uncertainty which so often manifested. Yet it wasn't just out on the trail that Ruby was altered, I pondered, there were visible changes from day to day too. As there also was for Winston and Millie. Here, they were kinder with each other, although boundaries were still maintained forcefully for the ever-insistent youngster. There was a greater sense of relaxation, their magnificent bodies shone with health, were soft and fluid and their reactions consistent.

There was also a greater level of cooperation between us all. Often I did not need to reach for a rope or a halter, I would touch a shoulder and they would follow. They would back out of my space if I even had the thought that they were too close. Words like 'connection' and 'closeness' were beginning to fall way short of the cord which linked us.

176

I should have expected that Ruby's reactions out on our first ride would be changed and that the balance in the herd was evolving. Why would they not be, when I had made such a significant shift within myself? How often had I written or spoken about the way in which horses respond to our inner stories? About how what we think, feel and believe dictates the energetic imprint which we have around us?

Like the angry gardener who had upset the delicate equilibrium of my home, I had no less been exuding the energy of my uncertainties and struggles over the past few years. In spite of 'knowing' all this I still got lost in the trance of my dilemmas. How different my presence must now feel for these three creatures as I am finding certainty, clarity and a contentment which ignites at a blink of their eye, a touch of a whisker, a glanced profile through my window. My love for these three creatures, and all their species, and for how they help me to *feel,* was beginning to surpass description.

50

Janet's Story

A disparate group

The four individuals gathered around me were about as different as they come: Janet, whose small stature belied an imposing energy; Pierre, a self-effacing, retiring man; Oliver, a precise, angular character who paid attention to every technical detail of the proceedings, and Isabelle, a wise soul nearing the end of her career who hugged anyone conveniently placed for her to do so and who quickly became the observant voice of compassion.

It was the second day of the programme which I had returned to the UK to deliver. I had not worked with any of the group the day before, nor they with each other. They were meeting the herd of two learning partners, whom they were teamed with for the day, also for the first time. Lotty, a confident, playful mare of four years old and Evie, a couple of years older and with a strong attachment to food.

'I didn't really get over my nervousness yesterday,' Oliver confessed almost apologetically as we discussed what they hoped for from our work together. 'I did try, though.' He went on to explain that he had been bitten by a pony as a boy and the memory still haunted him.

'And what helped you yesterday, Oliver?' I checked.

'Having a facilitator or a more confident member of the group nearby made me feel better. I know in my head that these horses are friendly, but I can't get it out of my head that they can also hurt!'

'I'm pretty nervous too,' offered Pierre before I could respond. 'I've never had anything to do with equines of any sort. They are just so big and I don't really know what to do around them. It helped me yesterday when your colleagues explained the horses' body language so I knew what they were feeling.'

'And how do you feel about being here?' I turned to Janet and Isabelle.

'No problem for me!' claimed Janet which surprised me because she was holding her shoulders high up around her ears, with hands thrust deeply into pockets.

'I rode when I was at school, so I'm feeling confident,' followed Isabelle. 'In fact I am wondering if I could fit one in my car when I leave.'

With two members of the group worried, and one who was but didn't own it, I would need to hold the process that day more closely than I usually might.

Forming

'I'll go first!' declared Janet when it was time to begin rapport building with Evie and Lotty.

'The task is for us to go in as a group today, not one at a time.' corrected Oliver sharply. 'We need to harmonise our collective energy, then when we are centred as a group we can join the horse herd and harmonise with them. That's the brief.'

'Yes but with two of us nervous I thought it would be better if we went in one at a time,' argued Janet.

When they looked to me for adjudication I gestured that they needed to resolve this discussion amongst themselves. Janet reluctantly agreed to proceed according to the brief and the four huddled together to establish a grounded and centred group energy.

179

As they prepared to move on Isabelle offered support. 'How can Janet and I support you guys who are less confident as we go into the paddock? How about if we pair up then you will feel like someone is watching your back?'

'That works well for me.' Oliver said warmly.

'Me too,' added Pierre.

Tension relaxed around the group and I noticed Lotty beginning to take an interest in them from across the green space.

'Are we all ready then?' asked Isabelle and I opened the fence up so they could enter.

A loose cannon

The two pairs hovered once inside the paddock, shoulder to shoulder. They whispered to each other and one pair peeled off to engage with Lotty and the other with Evie. My colleague and I positioned ourselves so we could shadow one pair each. I watched with horror as Janet, who was matched with Oliver, broke away without consulting him and began marching across to the far side of the paddock where Evie grazed quietly. Simultaneously Lotty came to life, perhaps stimulated by the fluctuation of human emotions, and began to canter around throwing in the occasional buck for good measure. She presented no risk, but Oliver did not know that. Isabelle stepped protectively in front of Pierre as the young horse came to rest before them. The two were soon ruffling her mane affectionately under the watchful guidance of my colleague.

In a second I reached Oliver. His terror was real.

'I'm shaking to my shoes.' he said as I ushered him out of the paddock. 'I know Lotty was miles away but I was terrified when she was galloping around.'

I called to Janet, who continued to stalk Evie, and then to Pierre and Isabelle, asking the three of them to join us. When

I opened the space for them all to discuss what had happened, Janet broke the silence defensively.

'I could see that Oliver was nervous so I thought I'd go ahead and smooth the water with Evie. Get her on side.'

I looked around at the other three members of the group. Oliver's look could have killed. 'Well I *was* really scared,' he retorted, 'But not till you walked off and Lotty started tearing around. You were meant to be watching my back!'

Pierre then turned to Isabelle brightly. 'Thanks for putting yourself between me and Lotty, it really helped. I loved it when she settled down so quickly and we were both able to stroke her.' The woman beamed with pleasure.

Twice is a pattern

'We're going to join your learning partners again to continue the session. What do you all feel needs to happen in order to build trust with them as well as to rebuild it between the four of you?' I asked.

'We all need to do what we have agreed to do, and consider everyone's needs, not just do what we want. We learned yesterday that unless we have faith in each other the horses won't have any in us.' Oliver spoke without hesitation whilst avoiding eye contact with Janet, who ground the dirt with the front of her boot.

They began to move across the paddock again. I shadowed Oliver and Janet so I could step in if necessary. They chose to continue with Evie and before long they were both fussing over her like grandparents might over a new baby in the family. It seemed as if Oliver might be relaxing a little. Evie seemed comfortable with her two companions and dropped her head to the pasture beneath. Like a flash, and against all instructions, protocol and guidance, Janet suddenly grabbed the left cheekpiece of Evie's head collar with a commanding: 'Come on, enough eating, let's go for a walk!'

'STOP!' This was no time for me to be subtle. Our 'house rules' dictated that it was unacceptable to force the horses to do anything, at any time, and Janet was also risking breaking her fingers. My command went unheard or unheeded.

'Janet, let go of Evie, now!' I raised my voice further.

She slid her fingers from around the leather strap and turned towards me pouting.

'I'm sorry for shouting orders at you, Janet. I don't like to do that unless I feel you are putting yourself, and others, at risk.'

'Oh! Was I doing that?' she retorted.

'You were!' chimed Oliver.

The situation risked deteriorating even further given the strength of feelings at play. 'Let's break for coffee and pick this up afterwards,' I said, forcing out a long deep breath from my lungs. I needed to calm down too and reflect on what to do next.

Half-way through the break, having regained my composure, I tapped Janet gently on the arm. 'Might we speak outside?"

In the farmhouse garden, far away from the good humoured buzz of the classroom I asked Janet to recall how she wanted to benefit from the programme.

She cleared her throat before responding cautiously. 'Er yes, alright. My boss told me I need to focus on the leadership side of things. My team isn't very motivated right now. He is thrilled with my personal sales figures, but the rest of the team don't do so well.'

'That is what your boss says. What do *you* say? What do *you* want from being here?'

The defiant look had dissolved. 'I... I... I don't know. I'm not sure now.'

'May I share what I saw happening this morning?' I asked. Janet nodded so I continued factually and without judgement. 'I saw you take control independently of the situation twice, in contradiction to the session brief, my later guidance and what you had agreed with your team mates. Can you bring some curiosity as to what that might be about?'

'I do like being in control,' she admitted after giving it some thought. 'I know that is one of the problems my team has with me. I don't want to be defined by my team though, I want to be seen to do well myself.'

'Say some more about that, Janet?'

'I want to know I can achieve things on my own, and show everyone else that I can too.'

I wanted to ask who she meant by 'everyone' but the group were now waiting for us at the edge of the field. It was a question which I felt also risked opening up more than we could deal with at that moment. So I simply clarified: 'As a leader in your organisation, your success is also measured by how your team does, I think?'

'Yes you're right, of course,' she rolled her eyes.

The foursome re-contracted for the rest of the day's activities. Isabelle paired with Oliver to give him more support and Pierre, who was increasingly confident, partnered with Janet. They began to settle as a team and the horses' level of cooperation increased as we moved onto leading and directing the herd, an activity in which we began to employ the careful use of lead-ropes to communicate intention to the horses.

Lotty, with Isabelle and Oliver's leadership, manoeuvred herself enthusiastically around the small obstacle course. Both humans gave her, and each other, attentive regard and clear communication. They were rewarded enthusiastically with a reciprocal enjoyment of the process.

At first, it seemed as if Janet and Pierre would enjoy the same level of success. Evie walked forwards with the lightest suggestion through the rope, turned left and right gracefully and only put her head down to eat when the temptation of the grass became too much. Hallelujah!

I celebrated too soon. Having completed one tour of the course, which was all that was requested, Janet stepped between Pierre and Evie, wrenched the rope from his hand and made to march away with the horse. As the word 'STOP!' passed my lips for a second time, Evie also had something to say and, swinging her head round, grabbed the sleeve of Janet's coat with her long teeth.

Self-sabotage

When I reached the woman she was clearly shaken.

'Are you hurt, Janet?'

'No, she just got my coat, that's all.' From the rip in the fabric burst a wad of white padding.

'Let's give Evie some space, shall we?' I showed Janet how to undo the head collar and the mare drifted away to graze.

'I feel stupid.' The woman looked downcast. 'Why did I do that when things were going so well? Why do I always mess things up?'

'We don't always understand why we behave as we do,' I replied gently. 'The good news is that often the simple awareness of a behaviour pattern can lead to change, without necessarily understanding its origins.'

'I just have to take over, it always seems like the best thing to do at the time. Then I sabotage things. For some reason it's irresistible. I just can't seem to allow anything to go well, or anyone else to be successful. I used to do it as a kid. I was always spoiling games or breaking toys. It never made me popular but guess what, I carried on doing it anyway.'

'You told me earlier that you liked to have recognition for yourself, rather than for the team…?' I brought her back to the present day.

'Well, that isn't really true. I think I was just trying to justify what I did this morning … I didn't cover myself in glory after all … deep down, you know what, I even sabotage projects I am solely responsible for. I can't even let myself succeed. It is a wonder that I have got this far.' She laughed weakly.

'You must be doing something right.'

'I've always brought the sales figures in I guess. That is usually what counts at the end of the day. Perhaps not anymore though.'

'What does success mean to you Janet?' I continued.

'Success means recognition and praise, more responsibility, a good feeling inside.'

As Janet said this, behind her Evie turned tail and walked away.

'Evie isn't convinced by that. I am not sure I am either,' I observed kindly.

Janet's gaze followed Evie as she drifted over to the rest of the group who were now standing waiting quietly in a huddle. The woman absented herself into thought.

Controlling through conflict

'Let's take it from a different angle. What do you gain from sabotaging your success?' I tried again.

'Ah, that is easier to answer. I get to blame other people for what has gone wrong. There is usually trouble too, a bit of a dust-up. I thrive on that. I was brought up with it. I find conflict more alive, more exciting, more productive. It's also easier to control a situation by wrecking it than blending in when it is going well. But I know all this, I've had counselling for years in the past, about how things were when I was growing up. The only way I got attention was by being naughty and being more destructive than my parents. I could write an essay about what I do and why, but that doesn't change the fact that I still keep doing it.'

'Change doesn't stick when the understanding is only in our minds, Janet. We need to feel the difference in our bodies. Once we get the felt sense of what the new, desired state is like, and it feels good, we can repeat it. There is still time today to be experimental, and see what it feels like to blend in when things go well, as you put it, and to share the kudos for that as a team.' I looked pointedly at the rip in her sleeve which Evie had left and said playfully. 'Maybe this can serve as a reminder?'

We returned to the group, and Janet related a summary of our conversation to the others.

When the work is done

During the next, final session of the programme Janet left the leadership of the team to Isabelle. Isabelle and Oliver completed their time with the horses by moving effortlessly around the arena with Lotty shadowing them, now and then pausing to pet and praise her and share their delight with each other. Then it was Pierre and Janet's turn. I hoped beyond hope that they would have a good experience.

Pierre took up a brush and began grooming Evie, who stood lapping it up beside him. Janet had placed herself about six feet away, her jacket placed on the ground with the torn sleeve on display. I could see her discreetly counting out her in and out breaths as I had shown her earlier, as a way of slowing herself down when she felt the urge to take over.

In a moment of pure spontaneity Evie, whom I could have hugged and kissed right there, tilted her nose towards Janet, before approaching. The woman laid a hand on the mare's shoulder, then a cheek on her flank. Pierre slipped the brush into his pocket and placed a stationary palm on Evie's other side, the three of them connecting as one being. Evie began to yawn and stretched her jaw, in total relaxation. I knew that the work for Janet was done.

Preparing to leave the arena some moments later, after the horses had been turned back out into the pasture, I noticed one of her colleagues pass Janet her jacket.

'That will be quite easy to mend I should think,' she offered.

'Oh, I won't be getting that repaired,' Janet replied. 'I will be getting it framed and hung on my wall.'

I hoped that over the next few months Janet's colleagues would be able to acknowledge her efforts to change as immediately as Evie had. And that perhaps they might also give her a little metaphorical nip on the sleeve every now and again, to keep her on the right track.

51

Perfection in Imperfection

June 2019

Grey skies over a soft steely swell saw me 'en route' back to France. A round trip passing through sadness and gladness. A strange process of leaving and arriving where each departure tugs and arrival brings rejoice. The privilege of loving people and places. In just a month I would be running my first residential retreat on the other side of the Channel, working at my own centre, with my own herd, in exactly the way I had always wanted.

There would be a small group on this first programme yet the to-do list I wrote later that day was overwhelming. Things which hadn't seemed important, suddenly were: the overgrown flower bed by the main gate, the weeds in the drive and hay-dust gathering on the eaves of the barn, the stains on the horses' bodies after lying in the mud, the cobwebs in the guest accommodation which renewed nightly, the creases in the sheets I had ironed twice already. Three weeks to go, and I was crushingly tired. And I had not even begun to prepare myself to lead the workshop which was surely the most pressing requirement of all.

Change of plan

Opening my emails one evening brought unwelcome news. Three of the people I was expecting to come were cancelling.

All for unconnected and understandable reasons. This left me with only two delegates both of whom were local. Despondency settled as I realised that the kind of programme I had planned was no longer possible.

Yet as I went about my chores the next morning I began to adjust my outlook based on this new information. The air had most certainly been let out of my balloon that was true. But then I began to chuckle at how absurdly, naively optimistic my plans were. I had underestimated what it would take to prepare the venue for visitors. I'd need three of me to be ready in time. Additional resources would be required in the future, that was clear.

I contacted the two remaining participants and they welcomed the opportunity to visit for private sessions instead of attending a group-based retreat. A solution which everyone was happy with.

I thought back to Janet and the tear in her jacket. She had developed a pattern of self-sabotage based on the need to control her environment. For her it was easier to do that through destructive behaviour rather than constructive. Perhaps I was not immune either to destroying what I was setting out to create. I was doing so by expecting too much of myself, once again. It seemed that my old achievement drive was still alive and kicking.

Harmony without control

Some of my stress as I prepared the site for the workshop was also caused by a desire to control. A drive to create something orderly. And nature, if left to its own devices, is not tidy. I had been despairing at the thriving crop of dandelions in my lawn, the nettles around my fence line, and birds nesting noisily where they were not meant to. There could be no tidiness here, no domination of the vegetation or the wildlife living within it. Nature was teaching me to coexist, how to find harmony *without* control. I was beginning to understand that, as far as my environment was concerned, order was to be found in a beautiful disorder, and perfection in imperfection. I wondered, might this apply also to ourselves?

52

Marie-Pascale's Story

Her eyes fell immediately on the form of the horses, framed against a backdrop of willows, oaks, poplars and ash. Marie-Pascale sighed deeply. A midwife, she had been signed off work due to stress some months before. For this first client session I was leading in France, I had thrown a simple tablecloth over my garden table, added a vase of roses and a jug of iced lemon water. The cobwebs fluttering in the breeze and the riotous lawn which attracted bees with its clover blooms, were part of the same soothing picture.

The herd sleeps

Millie leaned her weight against the fence, inquisitive to meet our new herd member for the day. Millie stayed alongside us as I led us into a standing meditation. I could hear her breath deepening along with ours as she fell into a light sleep. When I opened my eyes I saw that Winston and Ruby were also snoozing on all four feet. Millie joined them but lay down, front legs curled like a cat.

'Should we really disturb them?' whispered Marie Pascale as we entered the field.

'What would that mean for you, Marie-Pascale, if we did?'

'Oh, I would hate to do that! It wouldn't be fair.'

'That seems important to you so we will aim to *not* disturb them. To go a little nearer, but without interrupting their nap. Focus on your breathing, see if you can match theirs. If they become at all uncomfortable about our proximity, we will back up a little.'

Taking baby steps we inched closer. Far from being startled by our approach, Ruby lay down near Winston and soon he followed suit too. An event which is not unusual during working sessions, but not common either.

'Are they bored with me?' whispered Marie-Pascale. There was a worried wrinkle at the bridge of her nose. 'Should I do something they will find more interesting?' Her words suggested that she felt conflicted. A moment earlier there had been concern about disturbing the herd, now there was a desire to entertain them. I felt a confusion within me too.

'I'd like to be guided by the horses, to see what it's like to settle into doing what they are doing. How would that be for you, Marie-Pascale?' I continued.

'OK so what shall I do?'

I guided her to choose just one horse she could 'shadow' by again matching their breathing pattern.

'I will go with Millie. She seemed to like me the most. And she is the nearest.'

'Take yourself back to the meditation we did earlier. Get yourself into that grounded state again, then draw a little closer to Millie. Feel for an almost imperceptible 'Stop' sign, as you near her. This will be the edge of her personal 'bubble', if you like. You will have a sense of where it is. You might also feel tingling in your fingers, or feet, or gut. If she feels you are getting too close, she will tell you first by swishing her tail or putting her ears back. If you miss those cues she will probably stand up.'

Finding the edge of learning

Marie-Pascale moved forwards and rested about three feet away from the white pony and I smiled encouragement when she looked around to seek it. By this time Winston had stood

192

up to stretch, and returned to sleep, this time standing up. Minutes passed by and I noticed that Ruby was showing signs of tension in her body. She rolled onto her side and stood up, Millie followed suit. The three horses were now standing yet the mares began closing their eyes again. They shifted the weight from one foot to another getting comfortable.

'How are you doing?' I asked Marie-Pascale quietly as I leaned into her.

She startled me by throwing her arms up dramatically 'This is boring! It was fine for the first few minutes standing around doing nothing. But really, it was a long way to come to do it all day!'

The eruption threw me a little off balance. I registered however that the horses still rested which often they might not have done when a sudden fluctuation of human energy occurred nearby. Nor had they released emotion by licking and chewing. I guessed that the petulance seemed only skin deep, and that Marie-Pascale's reaction may have been because she was uncomfortably close to understanding what she needed to.

'What would you like to do instead of standing around, Marie-Pascale?' I asked.

'I'd like to groom Millie.'

Safe enough to sleep

I passed a soft brush to the woman but as she moved towards Millie the pony lurched to her feet suddenly and shook herself down. Marie-Pascale backed off. I got this strong feeling again of conflicted energy – a desire to 'do' and 'not do'. A need to be unseen and a need to be seen. I would have to follow the guidance of the herd again, who were still showing no signs of wanting to do anything other than staying inward. So I did nothing and observed the young woman hover nearby.

'I wanted something to happen!' She spun round, spitting the words at me.

193

'Something did happen. Can you reflect on it and tell me what it was?' I responded.

'I rested with the horses, stood near them. They all went to sleep. I was bored and then when I tried to groom Millie she shrugged me off!'

'And what sense do you make of it all, Marie-Pascale?' I invited.

'Well I suppose they were bored with me. Which is why they fell asleep.'

'I've got a different take on what happened.' I proffered. 'You see, in order for horses to sleep lying down, they need to feel safe. At least one will always remain awake in order to act as look-out. Just now, they all lay down and they all went to sleep. Does that knowledge change anything for you?'

Marie-Pascale's mouth opened and closed as if she was about to speak and decided not to. Then she asked, disbelievingly.

'Really? Seriously? So you are saying that they must have felt safe with me, before, when they were lying down?'

'That is what their behaviour could suggest, although I can't read their minds.'

'So then why did they stand up again? I suppose they stopped feeling safe, did they? Was that because I got annoyed?'

'I cannot tell you that, Marie-Pascale. All I can do is observe their behaviour and share what I see with you. It is for you to make sense of your experience.' Behind Marie-Pascale, who stood in pensive silence, I could see the herd beginning to come to life. The energy was shifting quickly, the right thing was happening.

'How would it be for you, Marie-Pascale, if that *was* true? If you being beside them made them feel safe, like when you started the session?'

She hugged herself, rubbing her ribs and then her upper arms as if she had just shivered.

'It would make me so happy, to think that. To believe they had been so comfortable with me. That they wanted nothing from me, other than my presence. That they didn't find me boring.'

As she spoke one of the herd yawned and stretched themselves back to life.

'Perhaps now is the time to go to them again Marie-Pascale?' I prompted.

They greeted her one at a time like a long lost friend, sweetly sniffing her hands. She stayed with them, her back to me, head and shoulders bowing towards them.

Presence is enough

'That was incredible,' began Marie-Pascale when we sat at the picnic table to close the session. 'I have lived for so many years with this belief that people won't like me. I work myself to the bone as a nurse, a daughter and a mother, just to feel like I matter. Then I lose interest because what I'm doing isn't making me feel better. I still feel lacking. When I switch off it feels like boredom but really I think it is frustration, all locked up inside me. I disengage because it all gets too much. That makes people uncomfortable, they distance themselves, triggering the cycle all over again. With the horses I experienced that same cycle: I disengaged from them, they then did from me at the beginning. But the big difference was they stayed with me until I found my way back to them. We were all able to come together again, without me having to give a pound of my flesh or jump through any hoops. All I had to do was stick with it.'

I closed the gates and watched Marie-Pascale's car heading up the lane. A craving for closeness to the herd drew me back to them, where I sat with a cool glass of minted water. Her cautionary words echoed. 'I don't have to give a pound of flesh.'

195

This woman had given of herself so much that there was almost nothing left. She would be visiting us again, our work was not finished. But for now, I turned my attention to myself, closed my eyes, breathing in the life which vibrated around the valley.

53

Holiday Lets and Heatwaves

July 2019

Even sitting still in the shade the sweat oozed out of my pores, soaking the scant garments I was reluctantly wearing. A blistering heat baked us. Lois, a German student participating in an international volunteering scheme, had come to help me for a couple of weeks. The horses cowered from the sun all day in the stone barn creating a backbreaking amount of muck to clear. Every hour they lined up expectantly so that I could turn the cooling hosepipe on them. They turned like figures on a music box to take the water on all sides. Afterwards I turned the jet on myself for temporary relief. So this is real heat. My prayers went to those in the world who live in these conditions routinely and my awareness of what global warming means sharpened.

Having postponed my plans to host therapeutic retreats that summer I advertised the on-site accommodation for tourists over the holiday period. I never fully appreciated what a deep clean entailed. Everything needed to shine and the linen stretch creaselessly across the beds. As fast as I swept away the dirt, more seemed to materialise. With two days to go before the arrival of the first guests it seemed that I was finally ready.

The invasion

'Pam, I think you should come!' Lois called from the lounge while I was washing up that night. We had been eating later and later due to the heat. It was already 10pm and having risen at 5am to profit from the cooler part of the day, my body needed to be horizontal. What on earth did she want?

Startled by her alarmed expression, I looked to the top of the window where she was pointing. A seething black mass moved against the dark wooden frame. As my brain tried to work out what it was, it began dispersing into the room. I put the light on. Flying ants, everywhere!

I watched with horror as more and more winged creatures crawled out of the woodwork around the window, the skirting board and even the ceiling beams, dropping from each tiny nook and cranny they could find to launch airborne into my house. There were thousands of them. The cupboard full of insecticide sprays and powders which the previous owners had left behind, and which I had not used, began to make sense. I grabbed the hoover in one hand, and against all my principles, a spray in another, scurrying from one entry point to another. The ants caught in our hair, the curtains, the carpet. Lois ran squealing to her bedroom. Why the ants had chosen to fly into the house and not outside where they were meant to be, I knew not.

The gite! I ran across the courtyard to find, even more bizarrely, a column of ants climbing the outside stone wall in order to enter the building under the eaves and fly in there too. I finished sweeping and hoovering in the house around midnight by which time the invasion had ended. Handfuls of ants had made it upstairs and I felt the need to vacuum my bedroom and shake out my sheets before climbing between them. The following morning I tackled the gite.

The ordeal repeated itself each night for six nights. At the same time, in the same places, the ants came in greater and greater volumes. At the hour of the day when all I needed was to sleep, I could be seen standing in a weary vigil waiting for them. By midnight it would be over, until the next evening ...

My guests, a French family from the South, took it in their stride. I supplied dustpan, brush and vacuum cleaner and they cheerfully volunteered to clean up themselves every morning. I wanted to kiss them they were so kind, not to mention that the husband bore a very close resemblance to George Clooney.

The way of things

On the seventh night as dusk fell I was ready for another biblical incursion. But through the window I made out a commotion in the air. Black shapes darted against the indigo sky outside. Dozens of bats of all shapes and sizes spun in a breathtaking aerial display. Tonight the ants had emerged where nature surely intended and for the bats it was time to feast. For me, it was time to marvel and remember nature's life-cycle, that everything has a place and a purpose and that, in the end, we all depend on each other. This was how it should be. I thought too, of my late brother, whose disparate obsessions included bat-watching (he had once even invented his own bat-detector). It seemed like he was with me, enjoying the spectacle.

54

Sophie and Winston

'I still remember the day that I met Winston. Every moment is etched on my mind as if on a living canvas.'

Sophie spoke poetically with a lilting French accent even though she had lived and worked in the UK for many years. She was one of my first clients when I began to integrate horses into my psychotherapy practice in 2008. Then she was a trainee psychotherapist herself, and went on to work full time in mental health services as well as raise a family, who were all young at the time of her first session.

A lasting impact

'Even before I arrived I remember being so excited, driving through the Cambridgeshire fens, expectant, hopeful, curious. Seeing all the birds and crazy hedgerows with their red berries and steam rising off the winter ground as the frost evaporated away. I knew it was going to be a special day, although I didn't realise how long the learning would endure.'

Seldom comes an opportunity for me to speak with clients a decade after they have worked with me, so I was excited to learn about Sophie's 'what happened next'. I was touched by the meticulous detail with which she could still recall the sights, sounds, scents and sensations of her experience.

She told me how she had first felt threatened by Winston's huge size and imposing presence, how it took the breathing exercises we had done to be able to relax enough to approach

200

him. Sophie remembered shadowing him in the field, offering nothing, asking for nothing, focusing on remaining mindful and in the moment.

'We were hanging out together and then suddenly the magic started to happen. This awareness of how intense my ability to *'feel'* was. And his powerful energy all around me. And then I realised that he had confidence in me. He made this funny noise blowing air through his nostrils then put his nose out to touch my hand. I was so elated!' Sophie then went quiet on the end of the phone.

'Are you still there Sophie?'

'Yes, sorry. I was getting lost in the memory of it all. I remember he pawed the ground with his front hooves and got down on the grass to lie down, I couldn't believe it! He looked even bigger lying there with his huge belly rising and falling as he breathed. Like this massive sleeping baby, so vulnerable and soft. This was the most significant part.'

'And what was it about seeing him lie down which had such an impact on you Sophie?' I asked.

What is stopping you?

'It was what happened next really, rather than the lying down itself. I remember telling you that I longed to do the same, to lie down and join him. Then you said it, the phrase which stayed with me. *What is stopping you?* And that was when I knew the answer to all I needed to know back then. I was the only one stopping me from doing anything. I was always holding back just that little bit. And I was doing it again then in the field.'

I let Sophie stay in silent recollection this time, to enjoy her memories.

'I remember you showing me where to sit so I would be safe,' she soon continued. ' I got down and stretched out flat on the ground staring up at the blue sky. It felt daring, but so beautiful as well. And I felt free. I didn't even care how cold the earth was beneath me. I just thought, I can do anything I want.'

'And how has that insight helped you since?' I asked.

'Whenever I notice that I am keeping myself slightly on the edge of events, or holding something back, or doubting that I can do anything, I just remember Winston and lying beside him that day in his field. It is strange because sometimes I still decide to withhold a little bit, perhaps at a heated meeting at work, or a social event where I am not comfortable. But the fact that it is an active choice to stay reserved is a completely different experience. I am doing it consciously in order to stay safe, not unconsciously because I am afraid. It is not the same thing at all.'

Sophie's description transported me back to our session all those years ago. Then, as a debutante in my new profession, I did not fully understand the potential of this way of working therapeutically. How deeply it would touch both my life and those I worked with.

My place in nature

'It was profound.' Sophie's monologue flowed with little prompt from me. 'I remember the intense feeling of inter-connection with Winston, with the whole of nature when we were lying down together.

'The sense of me being an animal, too. The relief of not having to use *words*. That we could both talk the same language yet say nothing. Accepting my unique, humble place in the animal kingdom has brought me a great sense of calm and perspective since. Especially when times have been tough. It has been particularly valuable these last four years while I have been working with families affected by the trauma of domestic abuse.'

'Can you say some more about that Sophie?' I explored.

'Nature makes us so whole, and in my job at the city hospital it is hard for me to access it. But I can simply close my eyes for a moment and be back in that field, feeling like a blessed part of the natural world. I sink into this space where I know I am not *separate*, not from anything. There is great comfort in that.

'When I find myself drawn into the horror of some situations my clients face, I imagine walking alongside Winston. It gives me strength. When I was at his side with each pace I got closer to being myself. That is how I stay in touch with who I am, so I don't get lost in the trauma surrounding me sometimes. I go alongside him in my mind.'

I put the phone down after we said our goodbyes and sat to savour the feelings of the moment. All these years my horse Winston accompanied Sophie, not just helping her but also the countless women and children she had in turn been assisting through her work.

Outside that evening, I leant my right cheek against Winston's side, close to where his heart lay beating. I wondered if he knew how often he had walked with Sophie and she with him. And I guessed that he probably did.

55

Beyond Words

After my call with Sophie I stood with Winston in the cool of the barn. I recalled the powerful experience I had with him when the nail was stuck in his foot. The feeling of our being so intricately connected, the wonder that he trusted me enough to help him, that he seemed to know exactly what I needed him to do. Then, when it was all over, how he wrapped himself around me so gently as I trembled.

I had learned already that I could communicate with my horses through my body. That lesson began with Winston eighteen years earlier when my mother was dying. He was six years old and as inexperienced a teacher as I was student. The only way he could make himself heard back then was with hooves, teeth and his half a ton set against me. The message was not kindly delivered but it launched me on a process of discovery.

That an imagined softness in my diaphragm, or pillar-like strength in my spine, could transfer an emotional state not only to my horse, but into my own way of being, was the lesson. Mastering breath control and the release of muscular tension furthered my ability to calm both myself and my horse, as well as releasing little by little the painful feelings I was clinging to. It took years to fully establish these techniques which helped me to influence both equine and human herds alike.

As my expertise progressed, it became irrefutable that emotions live even more strongly within our energetic body than they do in our physical one, and that they are contagious within and across species. But now, alongside Winston, my fingertips traced the edges of another piece of the puzzle.

Who am I to assume?

What if, when I believed myself to be communicating *'to'* my horse, the messages were not coming from me at all? What if, as I struggled with the pliers and Winston's injured foot, the 'instructions' had come from him to me, not the other way round? What if the images I received in my mind, let's call them thoughts, about what I had to do to moderate my escalating panic, had been his reassurance for me? Who was I to assume that I was the wise one, who initiated leadership from my own consciousness? What if it came, to me, from somewhere else?

When doing client work with the herd I had unshakeable confidence in their guidance. For over a decade they had never been wrong. I had read about animal communication and seen practitioners at work. I believed in what they did but never quite understood it. But now, something was opening up for me – the possibility that I may have been receiving intentional guidance from the horses all along. And if this was the case, what were the implications?

Sophie was not the first client to speak of the durability of the relationship she developed with a particular horse and how the inspiration continued regardless of the time and distance by which they were later separated. Was this simply their memory at work? Or something more sacred?

The nature of connection

I began to consider the possibility that, once a connection is made between one being and another, a pathway is opened up for that connection to endure in a way which defies the delineation of species, the passage of the years and the separation of the miles? I had got used to sensing the formless companionship of my loved ones who had passed. The quality of their presence was too palpable, too alive, to be only a memory. And with Zeus I had this sense of an ancestral timelessness which transcended the present moment, which I couldn't explain. Could it be that Winston was *actively* supporting Sophie at the times when she needed him?

The enormity of what I pondered began to cause the very plates of my world to shift. For if we humans are capable of distilling insight and guidance from the natural, unpolluted sources of wisdom within all living things … if time has no meaning and we are all, of everything, at one, at once … this changes the game completely. Perhaps we might begin to truly enrich our world, instead of destroying it. We might heal the pain which causes us to hurt and to fear and create the circumstances in which love can thrive?

56

Laurent's Story

The rains had fallen overnight, bringing relief and a delicious dampness to the air on the morning that Laurent arrived. There was a gentleness to the tall teenager which showed in his graceful way of moving.

'I'm trying to get an apprenticeship. I've failed one interview and with two more to go, Mum thought it would be good for my confidence to do some work experience. I'm sorry if it's a nuisance. I'll try not to get in the way.'

Laurent was the son of an acquaintance so it was not appropriate for me to work professionally with him. But he was a kind and unassuming boy whom I would have wanted to succeed, so I suggested that he help me on the farm for a couple of days. The horses would find a way, I knew, of teaching him what he needed to know.

I left him filling hay-nets while I went to pick out hooves, mix feed and distribute fly masks.

'Sorry, I've only done two,' he flustered on my return.

'No problem, Laurent, we are not in a hurry. Don't forget I've been doing this a lot longer than you have so I am quite quick at things. Let me know when you are done and we will decide what we do next.'

Six limp hay-nets lay on the ground nearly an hour later. 'Sorry, they don't look very full,' he mumbled.

'They are fine Laurent, thank you. Now if you could scrub the water buckets and refill them that would be great.' I handed him the scrubbing brush and showed him where the tap was.

Again, he disappeared for what seemed like hours, returning with a constant flow of apologies for his tardiness and general lack of skills.

I was beginning to see why Laurent was not succeeding at interview. In this new environment it was understandable that he felt unsure of himself as any person might, young or old. Yet none of my patient reassurance was heard and the more he apologised, the more his confidence diminished, if indeed he had possessed any at all when he arrived.

Finding a place in the herd

The strength of the developing heat meant that Winston, Ruby and Millie, however, were now rooted within the stone walls of the old cow shed which served as their shelter. There was one thing though which I knew would tempt them out.

'Sorry, I don't really know what to do,' stuttered Laurent as he held the hosepipe rather helplessly. 'How do I get them out here?'

'Don't you worry about that Laurent. Once the cold water starts gushing from the hosepipe they will come and show you exactly how it's done. Stay there on your side of the fence, you can lean over to reach them.'

Within seconds of the nozzle spluttering into life Winston's nose poked through the opening of the double barn doors, followed by his great brown and white form. The two mares came close behind. As was their routine, they made an orderly line, offering each flank, the chest then rump, in rotation, for the refreshing flow which was offered.

'Oh wow! That's amazing! They love this don't they!' It was the first time Laurent spoke without apologising. He was gleeful.

Every hour, on the hour, the teenager eagerly repeated the task. I thanked my stars for a spring-fed water supply which cost nothing. Between each equine shower, I showed him how

208

to collect different seed heads, plants and herbs from the pasture and garden which he could add to their feed buckets before he left.

'Same time tomorrow morning, then, Laurent?' I shouted as he climbed into his mother's car.

'Yes, please, if that is OK? And ... er ... thank you.'

I noted, with curiosity, that this was the first time that day Laurent had said 'Please' and 'Thank you', and that he had barely uttered the word 'Sorry' all afternoon.

The horses' help

The following day I got up early in order to finish all the basic chores before he arrived, so we would have more time to interact with the herd.

'Oh! You've finished the nets! Sorry, am I late?' he greeted me the following day.

'No, you're not, Laurent. I did them a bit earlier because I wanted you to have the horsemanship lesson I promised you, before it gets too hot. Is that OK with you?'

His attention was not with me, however, it had drifted to the welcoming committee gathered at the gate affectionately.

'Do you think they remember me?' he asked.

'Undoubtedly!' I smiled. 'They were grateful for what you did for them yesterday.'

Laurent chose to have his lesson with Winston, and I showed him how to put the halter on the horse and lead him out into the paddock.

'The first thing we need to learn Laurent, is how to stay safe. This means being able to ask Winston to move in and out of your space. It means winning his cooperation as well as his trust.'

I knew that if the teenager could learn how to confidently manoeuvre a large horse, an interview would present little problem. After Laurent mastered the basics of leading

209

Winston, who acquiesced politely to his requests, I set out a few small obstacles.

'Now see if you can guide him to walk a large figure eight Laurent, like this.' I walked out the exercise to demonstrate. Comprising two loops, the first going around one cone clockwise and the second around an adjacent cone anti-clockwise, it was a reasonably complicated sequence for a novice handler, but one which was familiar to all the horses.

By now the heat was building, the sun burnt through my hat onto my scalp. Every attempt to lead Winston around the cones ended in both human and equine being confused and I wondered if I had set too hard a task. Winston planted himself in front of the young man, ears pricked forwards in a clear question, 'What do you want?'

'I'm sorry. I'm making a mess of this. Sorry Pam. Sorry Winston!' Laurent despaired.

The horse's question went unanswered, so he took matters into his own hands, walking over to each cone in turn and stamping on them as if to say 'Will this do?' before marching off, taking the rope in Laurent's open fist with him.

'Sorry, he wasn't meant to do that! I hope he hasn't broken them!' exclaimed Laurent, whose confidence seemed to again be in tatters. I kicked myself.

All you have to do is ask …

While I was reassuring the boy a movement in my peripheral vision caught my attention. Ruby was making her way down from the corral towards us. She paused behind him, looked at me and then back at him.

'There is someone here asking for your attention, Laurent.'

He spun round. 'Oh! What shall I do?'

'Why don't you ask her what *she* would like you to do?'

I helped him to slip the halter off Winston and onto Ruby. With a light step the shining, copper mare made for the cones

210

and executed a perfect figure of eight, finishing her circuit at the side of the dumbfounded student. She touched him lightly on the forearm. Millie had drawn close and the two flanked Laurent as he stroked their noses and swatted the flies from their lashes.

'I don't really understand how that happened,' he said, bemused. 'I didn't do anything.'

'Did you ask her to do the figure of eight?' I queried.

'Not out loud. But I suppose in a way I did, in my head. I was saying please, please, please do it for me.'

'You know, Laurent.' I said. 'Horses have a knack of hearing our requests even when we don't speak. And they usually want to help. Humans too, on the whole. We just have to know what we need and how to ask for it. Usually with humans though we have to say it out loud!'

'Wow, really? Ruby can read my mind?'

Before I could answer, the horse shifted her shoulder away from us and looked up towards the corral, where the hosepipe and tap lay. 'She can,' I replied. 'Can you read hers?'

His puzzled look quickly melted into recognition. 'She wants a bath!'

The day continued as the previous one, interspersed with the hosing of the herd and foraging for their meal. Laurent found his place amongst them, through acts of giving and receiving. I hoped that these seeds of self-assurance would help him to ask for what he needed and show what he had to offer when it came to his interview and beyond. I heard some weeks later that he had been offered an apprenticeship to begin the following autumn.

Conscious healers

The exercise which Laurent was attempting to complete was one which Ruby knew well. It was something I did with her regularly to help maintain her physical suppleness and strength

211

following a history of pelvic injury. I could not know, of course, whether she completed the exercise on her own initiative, or whether she understood Laurent's inner pleas, or both. Either way she clearly 'volunteered' to help him, going out of her way to do so. Perhaps she recognised reflections of her young self in the boy, when she, too, was an unconfident learner anxious about transgressing the rules in a world she did not understand.

So often in the course of my work I have seen horses and ponies actively and consciously seek out a particular human to offer help. I believe that I have been chosen, too, by each of the horses in my life so that I may learn what they had to teach me. For every one of them I can remember as if it were yesterday, that first moment that I set eyes on them. When some kind of hook was thrown to draw me in.

The desire of horses to assist us consciously on our spiritual path represents the most profound truth about their nature. A nature whose depth we may never fully understand, but which I shall never tire of exploring, and by which I will never cease to be bewitched.

57

Savouring

Late summer 2019

The morning light plays amongst the translucent leaves of the young walnut tree beside me and steam is drawn skyward from the water meadow beyond. Drying herbs tied on the patio rail swing like fragrant metronomes, red fruits ripen on the raspberry canes, butternuts fatten and grapes sweeten as harvest approaches. Nearby in the small orchard pears, apples and peaches will soon be ready. Lettuce, cucumber and courgette are already gracing my daily plate.

Underfoot, wherever I roam in the teeming pastures, small creatures scurry, hop, crawl and squirm. Green grasshoppers two inches long jump, small snakes and lizards slide, butterflies, mason bees, honey bees, bumble bees and the huge black Normandy bees with midnight blue wings, are busy pollinating. But none of my fellow residents surpass the graceful hummingbird moths which hover at the honeysuckle and cosmos blooms, feeding on the nectar with their long slender proboscis.

I had not anticipated, before I came here, the impact which placing myself in this natural paradise would have on my way of being. It seems remarkable that I am provided for in this way. I better appreciate the intricacy of our ecosystem and the fine balance of our cohabitation, human with animal, insect, plant and flower.

213

And while I begin noticing, even more acutely than before, how often mankind wounds our world, by carelessness, ignorance or design, I am learning also what it is to deeply savour. To absorb with all my senses the taste of life itself, what it is to exist in each moment as it is lived, by the mind, body and spirit. From this consciousness my roots to the earth are strong and, like the water willows lining the stream below, my spirit can sway in the breeze, adapting to the changing emotions of my experience, leaning into the challenges, bending away from the worries, flexing to the confusions of relationship, the questions about the future, and returning back to centre where there is peace, stillness and strength.

Believing that I have everything which I need is becoming easier. The desire for more, to meet perceived lack through pursuit or purchase, is dispersing. The contentment brings liberation in a quiet kind of way. The need to hurry, to chase, to acquire, which drove my early career belongs now somewhere else. What I used to value, I realise I don't any longer. What was once a priority appears nowhere on my list. In the absolute simplicity of the natural world around me stands out the most important resource of all. The capacity for connection, with myself, with the 'other', the herd, the earth. The rootedness which results allows my emotional and moral compass to guide me around my dilemmas. I wonder, is this the gift of maturity, of the greying hairs increasingly more obvious when I look in the mirror, or the consequence of finding my right path to tread?

To whatever I might owe this settlement of spirit soon it will not only guide me but save my life.

58

The Wasps

September 2019

Ruby trod lightly down the horse box ramp into the lay-by at the edge of the forest. I saw in her a calmness and composure which, years ago, I had not thought were possible. Quietly and efficiently I prepared her to ride while she nibbled from the hay-net tied to the side of the van. I clipped my water bottle to the saddle, this would be a half-day ride, climbed up, settled into the seat and adjusted my stirrups.

'Show the way!' I called to my two friends who had ridden this trail before.

The parched stream beside us could barely be heard as we skirted the trees. The long hot months had taken their toll. The canopy colours were muted and we set up clouds of dust as we made our way along the stony track.

From above, the changes to Ruby's body since we moved to France were clear. Her shoulders, neck and rump had muscled and showed their power shyly through her silken red coat. Stretching my hand down I stroked her. My reins loose, my legs wrapping her roundness, my own physical and emotional self as supple and relaxed as hers. I was knowing the kind of harmony with this mare I had always dreamed of. We were at one, as one. I breathed in time with her as she walked. I was taken back to the time, as a young woman of 28, when I fell under the spell of a horse for the first time. I was riding a strong, chocolate brown Andalusian mare called Carabella through the Spanish Alpujarra mountains. One short week with her afforded me a glimpse of the soul medicine proffered by her species and of the irresistible draw of my destiny towards them.

The harmony of leadership

And now with my beloved Ruby the line between us was almost indistinguishable. Who was leading? Who was following? Where did I end and where did she begin as we passed through the dappled shade of oaks bending in acknowledgement above us? In this place of harmony, there was also balance – between us and within each of us. This, I sensed, is what leadership *really* is – a co-created symbiosis where one yields to the other, then vice-versa, as the way-finding ebbs and flows and where trust and respect work together in partnership. This is why horses are the best teachers of leadership on the planet – not because, as some of the theories explain, they are natural followers looking for strong direction from a dominant, focused alpha. But because they allow us, the student, to find this place of equilibrium within ourselves where we lose the need for control and gain the gift of presence. This place where leadership comes from an open heart and a clear sense of self, not from the badge that we wear.

A couple of miles into the ride the track began to climb steeply to the right, away from the stream and up into the deep shade of the forest. Up and up we went in single file with Ruby at the rear. The footing was difficult and with her neat hooves she picked her way amongst the gnarled roots and rocks as the path, barely a metre wide, wove through the trees.

Under attack

'I'm in trouble! Can you see what's happening?' My friend shouted suddenly. In front of me I saw her mare kicking out violently with a hind leg.

Before I could respond, her horse stepped forwards revealing a cavernous hole in the ground perhaps three metres in front of me. From it a cloud of angry wasps was swarming. Ruby and I were in even more trouble than my friend had been. The first in the line must have disturbed the underground nest.

I halted Ruby but the wasps were already homing in on us. In a split second I assessed my options. We couldn't turn round, it was too narrow, we were hemmed by trees both sides and the slopes anyway were way too steep. I couldn't get off for the same reasons and that would leave us more vulnerable to being stung. I could ask Ruby to back up, but she wouldn't be able to do that quickly enough given the terrain and that would leave the wasps between me and my companions who were disappearing ahead. There was only one way out of this and that was forwards over the erupting nest.

I squeezed Ruby with my seat. She hesitated but then, incredibly, stepped into the buzzing frenzy.

Images of what might go wrong sped through my mind. If I fell in this terrain I would be badly hurt. My panic was coming up. I wrenched my mind back into my body, back to Ruby. I had to stay calm, stay with her. Because everything, my life even, depended on *her*. Breathe Pam, relax your muscles.

'Go, go! Carefully!' I urged, giving Ruby the reins, resting my palms on her withers. I could feel her flinching as she took stings on her belly and flanks. She had picked up pace into a fast trot, her sides started to heave. Stumbling up and up we went, swerving in and out of the ancient trunks, pursued by the swarm. My knee banged into a twisted trunk, I clung on but lost my stirrups. Faster and faster she went. Still the wasps chased.

'All I have to do is stay in the saddle. And leave it to her. Stay in the saddle. Breathe. Relax muscles. Leave it to Ruby. Stay in the saddle.' I repeated to myself, hands pushing down onto her mane for balance, attention on my legs closed softly around her, staying close but not getting in her way. The track began its descent and ahead I could see my two friends emerging into daylight below.

We burst out from the forest track into a clearing bathed in sunlight. We were back on the riverbank. The wasps retreated into the woods, satisfied that we were not returning. I dismounted ungracefully, my knees doubling beneath me. My poor mare was coated in sweat, breathing heavily, and had small swellings where she had been stung. I checked her over, there didn't seem to be too much other damage and when she put her head down to graze, I breathed a sigh of relief.

'Ruby seems OK, but I need a moment to get over that,' I said. 'It was a close call.' The others got down too and we rested, quenching our thirst while the horses grazed.

When I felt ready we mounted up to continue on our way. But Ruby had barely taken twenty strides when suddenly her head dropped, lower and lower towards the ground and she began to stagger. I leapt to her side.

My mare's eyes were closing, her nose almost touching the track, and every muscle in her body twitched and shook. She swayed as if she might topple. Now I became the most afraid I had been since the incident began. I had never seen anything like this but I guessed she was in shock, which I knew could be serious for horses. Was it possible, too, that she could have an anaphylactic reaction? I didn't know. Whatever it was, she disappeared into an unconscious place, leaving me frightened. Would I lose her?

'I could ride ahead to go and get help,' offered one of my friends.

'Its a long way before you'll find a mobile signal never mind a house and how do we get a lorry down here anyway?' said the other.

'Well what about turning round – I could go back to our own transport, and find a way to come and pick Ruby up?'

'Then you'd have to go through the wasps,' I countered. 'And I think we need to stay together right now. Let's see if we can help her here.'

I loosened Ruby's tack, stood back and supported her as best I could with my presence. She was staying upright by some miracle, her bodyweight travelling from one leg to another, the huge muscles in her shoulders and rump trembling with a life of their own. I racked my brains, I knew from my professional training that mammals, including humans, discharge trauma through movement. Was that an option to consider? Time was passing and she was showing no change. It was worth a risk. I could be wrong, but I could also be right.

'Let's try getting her moving,' I decided, securing her saddle again and clicking a lead rope to her halter. If my mare was experiencing an autonomic reaction to what had happened this could be the best thing for her.

I tentatively asked Ruby to advance. She seemed to hear me and little by little began inching forwards one foot at a time. It was as if she was coming out of an anaesthetic, faltering, advancing, wobbling, righting herself. Head down, then up, then down again.

'Good girl, one more step. And another … now a few more …' I paused when she did, being careful not to ask more than she could give. Hoping beyond hope that she would be alright. Then her paces began lengthening, her chin gradually lifted. She was returning to me from wherever it was she had been.

A few miles along the trail and miraculously it was as if nothing had happened. For short stretches I mounted up to rest my legs and she was happy to carry me, and in several long hours we arrived at our destination.

219

Leading with love

Later that afternoon I sat with a cold beer in my garden. Ruby glowed in the soft evening sunlight and I absorbed the sight and sense of her. I knew that she saved me that day. Even while being stung, she did not buck, kick, bolt, slip or panic. She kept me safe. I had felt for a long time that I could trust my mare with my life and this was the proof. I can't quite define the emotions I felt as I watched her. Awe, admiration, gratitude, relief, pride, most certainly love.

There was also blinding clarity. The years of painstaking progress, when more than the occasional horse-owner sneered because I took so long to get her to accept the bridle and saddle or load into the lorry. I had allowed her to take the time she needed for the sake of our relationship, because that was what mattered. Now I truly understood why the quality of our partnership was so important. When the chips were down Ruby had put my safety above her own. When I asked her to step straight over the wasp nest she did it without question. I realised that riding is not what builds trust, it is when it is tested. That a bond between a human and a horse is built on foundations of love and of leadership, the kind which is borne out of care. That horsemanship is not about technique. It is about the wholehearted commitment to a spiritual journey through which we deepen our sense of ourselves, learn to be at one with all that is around us and strive to understand the other. Where we take responsibility for how we cause our horses to be and seek first to change ourselves. Where we meet them in their world and don't expect that they meet us in ours.

I had seen Ruby, Winnie, Millie, Dawn and Ellie offer healing to so many people. They rescued me, too, many times as well as the other horses who changed the course of my life – Carabella, Delilah, Gemma and Coop. But now Ruby had protected me physically too. For the devotion I had shown to my herd all these years, this was my payback.

220

I slipped quietly through the fence to join this mare who taught me not just how to be who I am, but to love that woman too. I offered the back of my hand in my habitual greeting, the one which says 'I give you my heart' and she pressed her muzzle firmly against my skin in acceptance.

59

Self-love and Compassion

November 2019

Soon I had the opportunity to return the care Ruby gave me. She stood uncomfortably beside my chair which I had placed beside her. The icy wind found its way through the old timbers of the barn, reminding me that it was winter outside. In the relentlessly wet weather she had developed an abscess in all four feet. The toxic shock experienced during the wasp attack may also have played a part in her condition. It was difficult to witness her shifting weight from one hoof to the other attempting to find relief. Now that the poulticing was done all I could do was keep her company while her herd-mates were out in the field.

That familiar voice began to whisper. You should have disinfected her feet more regularly. And noticed the symptoms earlier. Perhaps she is not getting the right nutrition. You must do more! You must be better! I set about sweeping the floor (again) and tidying the soft wood-pellet bed I had made for her. It was as if once I allowed anxiety to lodge in my mind, it wedged the front door open for all those old patterns of self-doubt to creep in. How easy it was to lose my ground and succumb to uncertainty and recrimination.

While my head filled with destructive chatter I noticed her move. Even though it hurt her to do so she took a small step away from me, then two. Tension was also beginning to show around her mouth.

Healing for us both

What on earth was I doing? I was meant to be helping her, but instead I was getting lost in my own world of self criticism and confusion. My diaphragm was as tight as a drum, in fact I was barely breathing at all and I had lost any sense of being in my body. I put the broom down, returned to my chair. I relaxed those constraining muscles around my eyes and held a soft focus. I felt into the space between Ruby and I for the energetic sense of her. Into the ache of unworthiness flowed calm and comfort. We are here and the situation is as it is.

Ruby sighed and began to yawn extravagantly, again and again. My own ribs followed her lead and we shared this moment of release and at-oneness. Her sore feet finally rested and she lay down to sleep. In the stillness I heard a voice within. I have done enough. I am enough.

It is with such grace that horses lead us gently to a place of self-awareness where forgiveness is possible, self-compassion takes the place of contempt and where they bring us into wholesome contact with our very soul. I pulled the blanket around my knees and stayed with her for a little longer. This was healing for both of us.

60

Waking up

December 2019

My friend's voice quivered slowly as she spoke to me on the phone, she in the UK, me in France.

'They've asked me what I want them to do … if … if it goes wrong. You know … during the operation. If I am going to be left paralysed from the neck down they want to know my wishes.'

The almost-silence told me she was crying. And I too.

'The thing is, I can't even contemplate living like that. Being dependent. Jessie having to look after me. I'd rather die. I think. Oh God, I just don't know what to do.'

I felt unprepared and unqualified for such a question. I didn't know what to say. The words came from somewhere inside me where instinct ruled over judgement. 'You only have one life, Grace. A choice to end it must be taken carefully, not now, not like this when you are under so much stress.'

Grace and I had been friends for many years, she was a little younger than me and was facing life-threatening surgery as a result of a benign yet currently lethal tumour which was growing in the spinal cord in her neck. After an unbearable few weeks, she was admitted to hospital and those who loved her had seven agonising hours to wait while she was in theatre. The call came that she was through it. I breathed again. At her bedside in London two weeks later I felt grateful to be looking at her, however poorly, before me.

Grace's battle to rehabilitate was not over, but she had travelled the valley of death and chosen life. 'I am so glad to simply be here. To have woken up.' She smiled weakly.

As the political warfare over Britain's place in Europe spread anger, fear and social rupture through the country of my birth, Grace's words were a salve. I learned to say each morning with the rising sun, 'I am so glad to have woken up.'

The gift of life

Grace reminded me how precious is the gift of life. The rest, when it comes down to it, is incidental. Whatever the outcome of the turmoil engulfing Britain, whether I would personally be allowed to stay in France, or not, surely this was all that mattered? That I woke each morning to welcome a new day, to savour it, to live amongst my horses, to give thanks and share the love which flowed so abundantly towards me. To notice every moonrise, each star and cloud which graced the sky, each raindrop which fell, each bird flying and bee collecting. To cherish every regard and glance from friend or stranger, each kindness, absence, presence, greeting and goodbye. Having faith in all that is, knowing I am blessed with all that's given so freely.

How could I know the importance of my friend's inspiring words? In just a matter of weeks, I watched images on the television screen of deserted streets and overwhelmed hospitals across the world. Borders closed, we were confined to our homes and, literally overnight, my business, like many others, was destroyed. This felt inconsequential as tens of thousands died, old and young alike, of the virus Covid 19.

Before emigrating to France I struggled to make my decision for months or perhaps even years. It was too daunting, too risky. I planned for a hundred and one different scenarios, anticipated every obstacle and turned myself inside out in an attempt to answer the fundamental question at the core of my dilemma: 'Will I be happy?'

The way in which global events unfolded, barely a year after I moved, could not have been predicted. I was, of course, asking myself the wrong question. The right one would have been easier to answer: 'Whatever happens, will I still have the capacity to find joy in my situation?'

Captive with the herd

I cannot leave my property unless it is to shop once a week or to take exercise. My younger brother is staying with me so at least I have some human company. I sit in the garden and watch the herd feed off their hay contentedly. Winston moves away and walks as if wearing heavy wellington boots on his hind feet, lowering his back end and stepping high with each back toe. A sure sign he is about to lower himself to the ground to roll. Once down, legs curled under him like a cat, he begins by rubbing an itchy spot on his tummy, rocking forwards and back, then flips to one side and the other, wriggling in the earth with considerable agility. Millie, the most hedonistic of the three, follows his example, grinding her mane, face and neck into the dirt, blowing air out through her flaring nostrils and throwing a sandstorm of dust into the air as she gets up.

The two mares now come together and begin grooming each other, nibbling manes, necks and shoulders, reinforcing their attachment. Winston politely moves Millie on and takes her place with Ruby. One after another they peel away, walking up to the water trough, then taking shade under the trees as the early Spring heat finds its form. Above me buzzards circle and screech. A nearby field has been ploughed and soon they will descend in sweeping spirals to feed on what they can find. A heron glides down from on high, its wings stretched wide like a ballerina's arms in that exquisite moment before she drops

226

into a curtsey. The bird crosses my field of vision, riding the air, ready to fall as lightly as a feather to the riverbank below.

Confined here, with nowhere to go, no work to call me, no visits to make, people to see or appointments to keep, my world has become so much smaller yet simultaneously so much more vast. How much there is to see, to feel, to understand, to love, to cherish.

I am so glad to have woken up this morning. To see the sun rise again. To savour all that is existence. To live in this beautiful place which I call home. Under the clear blue sky, void of aircraft trails, time is no longer counted. I am able to sink into the infinity of presence as the herd has taught me. My human agendas suspended, I am finally, exquisitely, attuned to the spirit of the horse.

Acknowledgements

My deepest gratitude goes to the many people who have come to learn in the heart of the herd, without whose courage this book would not exist. In particular my thanks to those of you who talked to me about your experiences with the horses and who have contributed so wisely to this narrative. To the characters of Grace and Jessie, whose love knows no equal, you inspire every day with your courage, heart and hope.

Thank you to my friends and family, to Justin for bringing his depth, emotional integrity and intellectual rigour to his reading of the final draft, to Janet for proofreading so meticulously, and to Emily for gifting the use of the stunning photograph on the front cover, taken one happy, shiveringly cold daybreak in the hills of Wiltshire. I would like to acknowledge, also, the talent, wisdom, love and friendship of the fellow professionals I work with and learn from every time (you know who you are!) and everyone at Suddene Park Farm, and Sue, who share their horses so generously.

For the amazing, inspiring, humble and most kind of humans, Stephanie Zia of Blackbird Books, who helped me discover, and let me keep, my confident writer's voice, thanks are not enough. She is the unseen force, the silent voice, concealed within every Blackbird book and if you read them all you will no doubt hear it too.

And finally, for the horses in my life, past and present, with their love, presence, forgiveness, affection, inspiration and gentle guidance I am blessed. They can't read this but of course, as you know, they don't need to.

Dear Reader,

I hope that you have found as much joy, comfort, inspiration and pleasure in reading *The Spirit of the Horse* as I did in writing it. Completed during 2020 when all our lives were turned upside down, the book, and the way it connected me to all that nurtures, became an anchor and a safe place. May it have been the same for you and may the characters within the pages, both equine and human, have touched your hearts as they touched mine.

In an age where algorithms and public 'likes' can make or break a book, it would be helpful if you were able to leave a constructive review of *The Spirit of the Horse* through one of the well-known retailers: Goodreads, Waterstones, Amazon, Foyles, for example. I read all reviews and it is good to know what you liked or didn't like and how *The Spirit of the Horse* has spoken to you.

If you would like to find out about attending one of my retreats or workshops, or receive remote or face to face coaching, therapy or mentoring, please refer in the first instance to my website www.pambillinge.com. If you are interested in exploring how horses could transform your organisation then you will find more information about that side of my work on www.equestlimited.co.uk. I can also be contacted via these websites or my Facebook pages if you would like to share your own horse story with me.

With nature's blessings

Pam